# Scaling Preservice Training in Comprehensive Contraception and Abortion Care and Research across Ethiopia

*A Case Study of a Five-Year Project with Schools of Medicine and Midwifery*

Solomon Worku Beza, Bekalu Mossie Chekol, Mengistu Hailemariam Damtew, Munir Kassa Eshetu, Azeb Tamrat Hailemeskel, Kathleen Ludewig Omollo, Elizabeth Randolph, Berhanu G. Gebremeskel, Tamrat Endale, Yolanda Smith, Daniel Rivkin, and Janet Hall

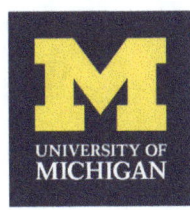 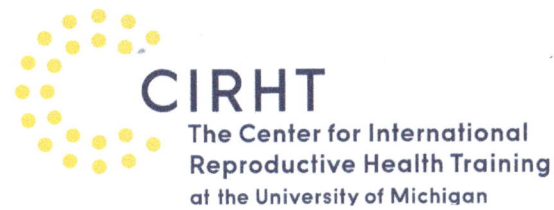

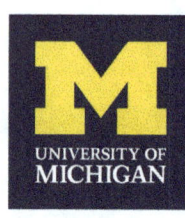 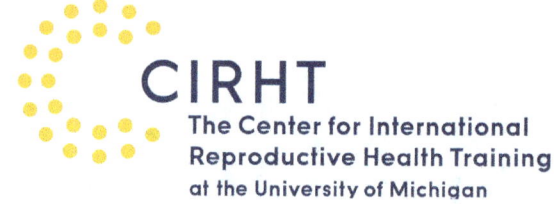

Copyright © 2019 by Regents of the University of Michigan
Some rights reserved

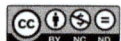

This work is licensed under the Creative Commons Attribution-NonCommercial-NoDerivatives 4.0 International License. To view a copy of this license, visit http://creativecommons.org/licenses/by-nc-nd/4.0/ or send a letter to Creative Commons, PO Box 1866, Mountain View, California 94042, USA.

Published in the United States of America by
Michigan Publishing

ISBN 978-1-60785-567-5

# Contents

| | |
|---|---|
| List of Figures | iv |
| Acknowledgments | v |
| Acronyms | vii |
| Executive Summary | ix |
| | |
| Background | 1 |
| Framework | 3 |
| Implementation | 5 |
|     Selection of the Schools | 5 |
|     Administrative Considerations | 5 |
|     Timeline | 7 |
|     Education Program | 7 |
|     Clinical Service Program | 15 |
|     Research Program | 20 |
|     Faculty Development Program | 27 |
|     Monitoring and Evaluation | 30 |
| Transition | 34 |
| Outcomes | 35 |
|     Overall | 35 |
|     Education | 37 |
|     Clinical Service | 40 |
|     Research | 45 |
|     Faculty Development | 46 |
| Lessons | 48 |
|     Overall | 48 |
|     Education | 49 |
|     Clinical Service | 49 |
|     Research | 49 |
|     Faculty Development | 50 |
| | |
| Conclusion | 51 |
| References | 53 |

## Figures

| | | |
|---|---|---|
| Figure 1 | Strategic Vision for UM-CIRHT, Developed in 2015 | 2 |
| Figure 2 | Core Programmatic Areas of UM-CIRHT Framework | 4 |
| Figure 3 | Location and Attributes of Partner Schools | 6 |
| Figure 4 | Timeline of Project Milestones and Key Events | 8 |
| Figure 5 | FP/CAC Sessions for Partner Schools as Defined in the Course Syllabi | 10 |
| Figure 6 | Research Milestones for Investigators | 22 |
| Figure 7 | M&E Approach of UM-CIRHT Framework | 32 |
| Figure 8 | Student and Resident Enrollment across Partner Schools by Graduation Year | 38 |
| Figure 9 | FP/CAC Assessments Conducted across Partner Schools, February 2017–June 2018 | 39 |
| Figure 10 | Safe Abortion Services by Trimester across Partner Schools, September 2015–July 2018 | 41 |
| Figure 11 | LARC Use by Trimester, September 2015–July 2018 | 42 |
| Figure 12 | PPFP Services across Partner Schools, August 2016–July 2018 | 43 |
| Figure 13 | PAFP Services across Partner Schools, August 2016–July 2018 | 43 |
| Figure 14 | Research Milestones Progress across Partner Schools, June 2015–July 2019 | 46 |
| Figure 15 | Faculty Development Training across Partner Schools, July 2014–July 2018 | 47 |

## *Acknowledgments*

The Center for International Reproductive Health Training at the University of Michigan (UM-CIRHT) would like to express our gratitude to the faculty, staff, and leadership of the following institutions:

- Adama Hospital Medical College
- Addis Ababa University
- Bahir Dar University
- Debre Tabor University
- Haramaya University
- Hawassa University
- Jimma University
- Mekelle University
- University of Gondar
- University of Michigan

Our sincere thanks go to all the trainees, medical students, midwifery students, interns, and OBGYN residents who participated in this pioneering program and willingly provided their feedback through surveys and interviews.

This case study would not have been possible without the input of each of our 19 interviewees, who generously donated their time and insight, providing the basis for the content of this report: Mulat Adefris, Bekalu Assamnew, Solomon Beza, Yibrah Berhe, Abiy Mergia Bulto, Amanuel Desta, Tamrat Endale, Munir Kassa Eshetu, Lia Tadesse Gebremedhin, Tsigereda Getachew, Yemisrach Getiye Tadesse, Mengistu Hailemariam, Azeb Hailemeskel, Janet Hall, Olivia Hannosh, Ephrem Lemango, Amare Mezmur, Bekalu Mossie, and Meghan Obermeyer. Their patience and cooperation were invaluable to the development process.

We are very grateful to the Ministry of Health of the Federal Democratic Republic of Ethiopia for its unwavering commitment to providing family planning and comprehensive abortion care to the women and girls in Ethiopia. The invaluable support and leadership from the ministry created a conducive environment without which the preservice integration program at all nine partner schools would not have been possible. We feel very fortunate to have been the ministry's partner in this work.

Finally, we express our heartfelt appreciation to Senait Fisseha, MD, JD, professor of obstetrics and gynecology at the University of Michigan, who initiated this project in 2014 as founder and first executive director of UM-CIRHT. We remain forever grateful for her vision and continued support to improve the lives of women and girls around the world.

Financial support for this project was provided through a grant awarded to UM-CIRHT from an anonymous donor.

The authors appreciatively acknowledge the editorial support of Michigan Publishing.

## Acronyms

| | |
|---|---|
| **CAC** | comprehensive abortion care |
| **CARD** | clinical and academic research director |
| **CARE** | comprehensive abortion and reproductive education |
| **CBE** | competency-based education |
| **CED** | chief executive director |
| **CUGH** | Consortium of Universities in Global Health |
| **D&E** | dilation and evacuation |
| **DHS** | demographic and health survey |
| **EBM** | evidence-based medicine |
| **EMA** | Ethiopian Medical Association |
| **EMWA** | Ethiopian Midwives Association |
| **FIGO** | International Federation of Gynecology and Obstetrics |
| **FINER** | feasible, interesting, novel, ethical, relevant |
| **FMOE** | Federal Ministry of Education |
| **FMOH** | Federal Ministry of Health |
| **FP** | family planning |
| **HMIS** | Health Management Information System |
| **ICFP** | International Conference on Family Planning |
| **ICM** | International Confederation of Midwives |
| **IUD** | intrauterine device |
| **LARC** | long-acting reversible contraception |
| **MCH** | maternal and child health |
| **M&E** | monitoring and evaluation |
| **MOU** | memorandum of understanding |
| **NMEI** | New Medical Education Initiative |
| **OBGYN** | obstetrics and gynecology |

| | |
|---:|:---|
| **OPD** | Outpatient Department |
| **OSCE** | objective structured clinical examination |
| **PAFP** | postabortion family planning |
| **PAL** | peer-assisted learning |
| **PDCA** | plan, do, check, act |
| **PI** | principal investigator |
| **PPFP** | postpartum family planning |
| **PREPSS** | Pre-Publication Support Services at the University of Michigan |
| **PWHER** | Program on Women's Healthcare Effectiveness Research |
| **QI** | quality improvement |
| **RAC** | research advisory council |
| **RH** | reproductive health |
| **SDG** | sustainable development goals |
| **SRHR** | sexual and reproductive health and rights |
| **UM-CIRHT** | Center for International Reproductive Health Training at the University of Michigan |
| **VCAT** | value clarification and attitude transformation |

## *Executive Summary*

Access to quality family planning and safe abortion services has been recognized worldwide as an essential element of public health policy necessary for achieving gender equality and women's empowerment in developing countries. Yet unmet need for contraception, unintended pregnancies, and deaths from abortion-related complication persist. To address this fatal imbalance, more health professionals are needed with the skills to deliver effective family planning (FP) services, safe abortion, and other comprehensive abortion care (CAC).

The Center for International Reproductive Health Training at the University of Michigan (UM-CIRHT) was founded in 2014 to partner with educational institutions in developing countries to strengthen the human resources for FP/CAC. UM-CIRHT utilized a preservice approach integrates FP/CAC into undergraduate and postgraduate curricula to ensure graduates acquire the skills they need before beginning their clinical service.

In July 2014, UM-CIRHT commenced a five-year project to scale preservice training in FP/CAC across Ethiopia. The project began with medical education and OBGYN residency programs at nine partner schools, revising curricula and strengthening FP/CAC education by providing resources and incorporating hands-on methods. In July 2016, midwifery programs at eight of the nine partner schools were added to the project. UM-CIRHT developed a theoretical framework for its four program areas: education, service provision, research, and faculty development. Interventions such as the opening of model FP clinics—called Michu (the Amharic word for *"comfort"*) clinics, where students could rotate and receive experience in woman-centered reproductive health care—were successful in improving quality and exposure of both preservice education and community access to these services.

While implementation was focused on FP/CAC topics, there was significant spillover into other departments and schools within the partner institutions. Other departments saw the value of preservice education and restructured their programs to shift more training into the undergraduate programs. Research trainings were open to all faculty, and researchers were required to form interdisciplinary teams. Education as a whole was greatly strengthened, specifically in simulation training, due to significant improvements to simulation lab infrastructure and faculty engagement. These system-level changes expanded the program's impact, increasing the likelihood of its sustainability.

In August 2018, the project transitioned to the Federal Ministry of Health (FMOH), solidifying the country's ownership of the project and validating the government's commitment to its sustainability. While keeping to the overall mission of educational capacity building, the FMOH aligned implementation with national priorities, integrating it with the overarching national vision to sustain the benefit of the investment beyond the end of this project.

# Background

Access to quality reproductive health care empowers girls and women to shape their lives and determine their futures. Sexual and reproductive health and rights (SRHR) have been recognized worldwide as an essential component for ensuring healthy lives and achieving gender equality. These shared values are reflected in two of the United Nations' sustainable development goals (SDGs) for 2030.[1] Within SDG 3, *"ensure healthy lives and promote well-being for all at all ages,"* there is a target to *"ensure universal access to sexual and reproductive health-care services, including for family planning, information and education, and the integration of reproductive health into national strategies and programmes"* (SDG 3.7). Similarly, within SDG 5, *"achieve gender equality and empower all women and girls,"* there is a target to *"ensure universal access to sexual and reproductive health and reproductive rights as agreed in accordance with the Programme of Action of the International Conference on Population and Development and the Beijing Platform for Action and the outcome documents of their review conferences"* (SDG 5.6).

The unmet need for modern contraception in developing countries affects 214 million women of reproductive age.[2] There are an estimated 73 million unintended pregnancies per year in developing countries, of which 49% end in induced abortion.[3] Over 22,800 women die each year from abortion-related complications.[2] In order to address this, more health professionals are needed with the skills to deliver effective family planning services, safe abortion, and other comprehensive abortion care.

UM-CIRHT was founded in 2014 to strengthen the human resources for FP/CAC by including it in the undergraduate and postgraduate curriculum in the preservice period, before health professionals begin their clinical service. In partnership with medical, nursing, and midwifery schools, UM-CIRHT works to ensure that graduates have the knowledge, appropriate attitude, and practical skills to meet the needs of patients and communities. With a mandate covering countries across Africa, UM-CIRHT seeks to reduce maternal mortality and morbidity from unsafe abortion by introducing the skills and culture for FP/CAC early in trainees' learning (see figure 1).

The preservice education approach UM-CIRHT uses is based on a successful project launched in 2011 to integrate FP/CAC into medical education at St. Paul's Hospital Millennium Medical College (SPHMMC) in Ethiopia.[4] That project involved some of the same team

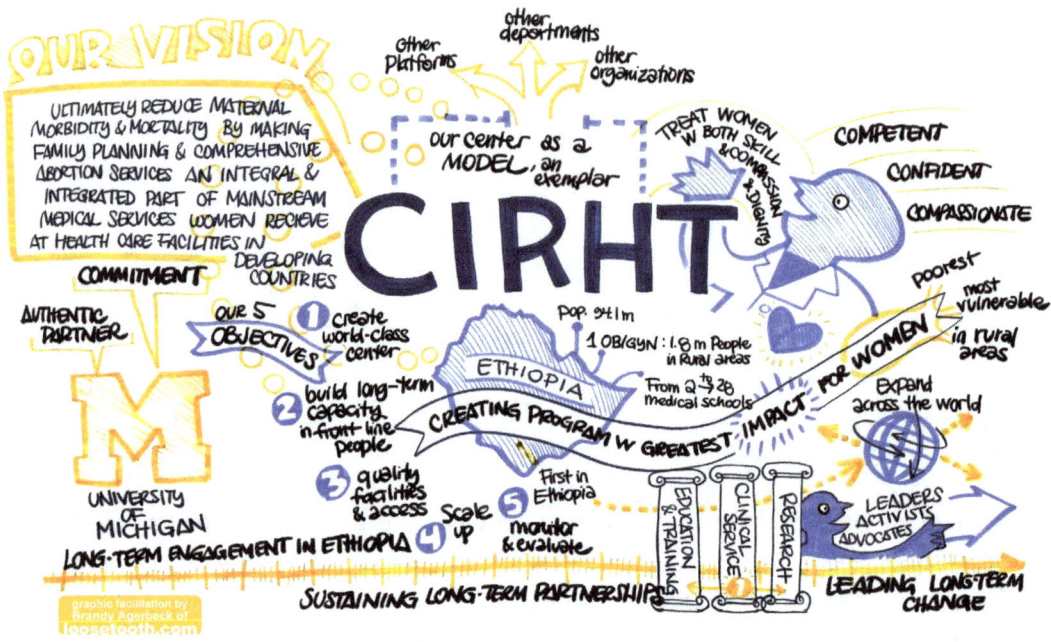

**Figure 1.** Strategic Vision for UM-CIRHT, Developed in 2015

members and was led by the founding director of UM-CIRHT, Professor Senait Fisseha. This project implementation began by expanding that model to nine additional schools and colleges in Ethiopia.

In recent years, Ethiopia has made impressive strides in reproductive health. The maternal mortality ratio fell from 1,250 per 100,000 births in 1990 (one of the highest in sub-Saharan Africa) to 412 per 100,000 births in 2016, a decline of 67% between 1990 and 2016.[5, 6] Women in Ethiopia today have an average of 4.5 children, about 2 children less than the average reported in the 1990s. The decline is mainly due to the effort of the Federal Ministry of Health, which has created policies and availed resources to further the aim of reproductive health access for all. Despite this progress, there are still significant gaps that lead to unmet need for contraception, unsafe abortions, and maternal morbidity and mortality. One contributing factor was insufficient FP/CAC training in traditional education programs for medical and midwifery students, who were subsequently unable to provide these services once they entered the workforce.

This retrospective case study examines a five-year project scaling preservice training of FP/CAC across nine Ethiopian schools of medicine and midwifery beginning in July 2014. It aims to capture lessons learned from implementing the framework and share them with other schools and health ministries planning to strengthen FP/CAC preservice training. This case study is based on semistructured interviews conducted in July–December 2018 with 19 individuals who held faculty roles in the partner schools or staff roles with the UM-CIRHT team in Ethiopia or Michigan. It also draws from document analysis of internal project files from across the full project period and participant observation by the case study authors, who were each involved in various stages of implementation.

- For the content, first UM-CIRHT convened a panel of experts from the partner schools, the FMOH, and the Federal Ministry of Education (FMOE) to review the curriculum and in some cases revise it to increase the duration of exposure to FP/CAC. This was harmonized with the national curriculum. Second, representatives from the panel developed a course syllabus for FP/CAC, as well as case studies and standard lecture slides. Some new resources were developed through a multimedia resources boot camp, and supplemental materials from existing free public resources were also collected.
- For the delivery, UM-CIRHT led faculty development workshops on clinical skills teaching; knowledge and skills assessment, including item development and objective structured clinical examination; competency-based education; and simulation-based training, as well as workshops for students on peer-assisted learning. The workshops focused on strengthening faculty as effective educators. Specific workshop topics and duration were tailored to the needs of each partner school based on the interests and schedules of faculty.
- For the assessment, UM-CIRHT facilitated standardization of student and resident logbooks across the schools and trained faculty in various learner-assessment methods for written and hands-on exams.

## Content

### Reviewed and Harmonized Curricula

The curriculum review focused on ensuring that the FP/CAC components were competency-based. Competency-based education (CBE) prioritizes clear learning outcomes, and the methods of teaching and assessment are developed in alignment with these outcomes. To assure CBE, core competencies need to be defined.

One of the first activities UM-CIRHT undertook was the collection of all the medical school curricula, followed by a thorough revision of the FP/CAC areas to standardize, strengthen, and clarify competencies and learning objectives. This was accomplished as a group, with representatives from each partner school participating in the harmonization, revision, and integration of the medical school curriculum. Representatives from the FMOH's human resources directorate also joined the discussion.

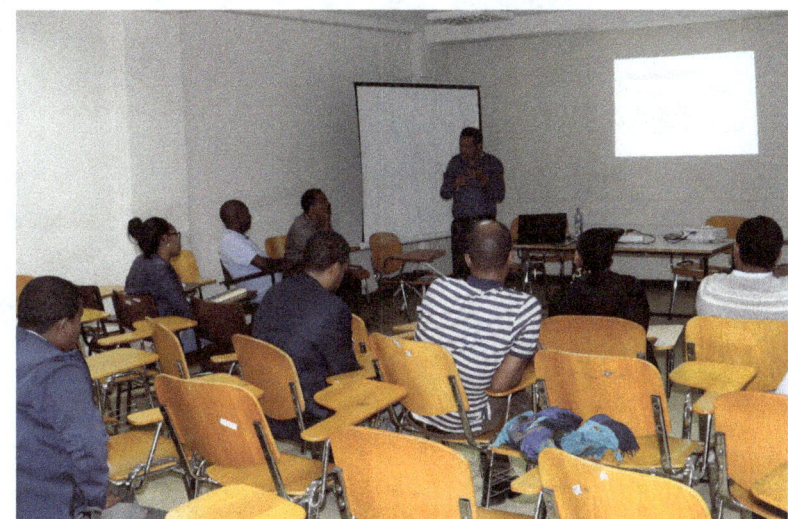

Faculty Curriculum Training

The midwifery curriculum review took a different approach. One midwifery faculty leader shared, *"Midwives mainly focus on attending deliveries as well as giving immediate newborn care for the babies. If there were more of them in every health facility, in addition to delivery work, they could counsel and advise on family planning services. With UM-CIRHT's assistance, we can share experiences and skills, creating benchmarks and best practices. I think that will help us motivate students and allow them to bring innovative ideas [for] bridging the gaps in health care that we may find."*

For the midwifery curriculum, the FMOH already had a standard curriculum that included FP/CAC. The baseline assessment revealed gaps in the awareness and delivery of those FP/CAC competencies, and how the schools chose to implement these topics varied significantly. To address this, the project used an approach similar to that used with the medical schools, focusing on revision of the syllabi and course materials.

When the UM-CIRHT project started, only three of the partner schools had active OBGYN residency programs: Addis Ababa University, Jimma University, and the University

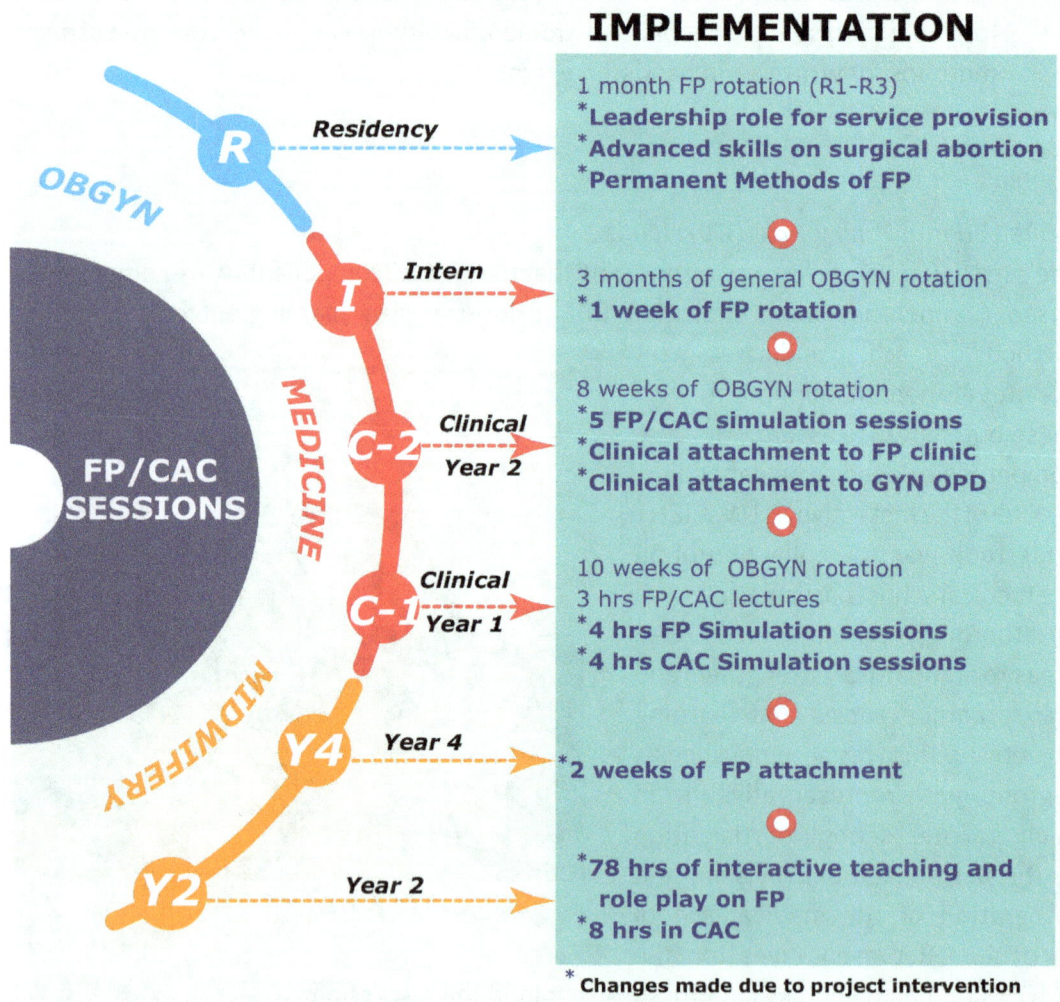

Figure 5. FP/CAC Sessions for Partner Schools as Defined in the Course Syllabi

of Gondar. During the course of the project, UM-CIRHT supported five other partner schools in formulating their OBGYN residency curricula, meaning only one partner school did not have an OBGYN residency program by the end of the five-year project.

*Created Course Syllabi*
Once the curriculum was revised to address the gaps that had been identified, UM-CIRHT brought faculty from each partner school together through central workshops to develop course syllabi for both FP and CAC. These syllabi became the core reference documents used across the schools to ensure standardization. Figure 5 shows the FP/CAC educational sessions for each program (OBGYN, midwifery, MD) as defined by its course syllabus.

*Developed New Learning Materials through a Faculty "Boot Camp"*
The next step was to address the identified gap of access to adequate supporting educational materials. UM-CIRHT decided to use videos, a flexible and cost-effective medium for educating large numbers of students that also supports self-learning. Videos also enable faculty with the means to implement new and innovative ways of teaching, like using a flipped-classroom model. In order to provide materials relevant to the local context, a small group of faculty participated in an intensive workshop, or *"boot camp,"* in November 2016 to produce their own video lectures; UM-CIRHT invited OBGYN faculty from each of the partner medical schools to the three-day event. Faculty came prepared with draft lecture slides, which went through a rapid peer review and then were recorded on video. The boot camp covered the concept of the flipped classroom, as well as principles of e-learning and instructional design, cognitive processes in multimedia learning, editorial and visual style guides, and production of engaging slide presentations and audio and video materials. During the boot camp, video lectures were created for different topics: short-acting methods of contraception, intrauterine devices (IUDs), contraceptive implants, postpartum family planning (PPFP), permanent and emergency methods of contraception, counseling, and CAC.

Boot camp attendees were able to develop skills in e-learning resource production, thereby enabling the continuation of locally produced multimedia resources. After postproduction editing, all resources developed at the boot camp were distributed to students at all partner schools and posted publicly on the UM-CIRHT website.

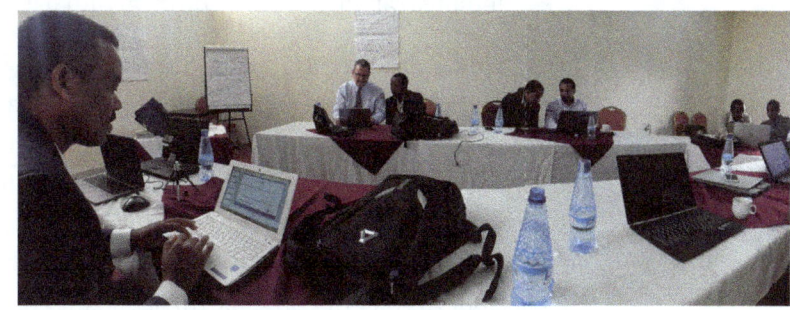
**"Boot Camp"** Presentation Preparation

*Curated Existing Supplemental Learning Materials*
Faculty and students requested paper and electronic resources to support the syllabi. Hard copies of textbooks were purchased and distributed to each school. Electronic resources were collected in partnership with library and information technology specialists, who

searched for materials on various reproductive health topics. Materials collected included electronic midwifery textbooks from an in-country partner as well as Open Michigan at U-M and other collections of open educational resources or freely available materials. In total, over 2,000 materials were organized into six collections and distributed to the schools. As internet connectivity can be unreliable, UM-CIRHT supported each school in setting up a platform that enabled students to access electronic resources without internet access. The same materials were also posted on a public website maintained at U-M.

### Delivery

#### Built Capacity and Awareness for Competency-Based Education

The various capacity-building workshops and trainings were intended for faculty who teach undergraduate medical students to acquaint them with the revised OBGYN curriculum and prepare them to use the teaching and assessment methods included in the curriculum. Similar workshops were provided for midwifery faculty to enhance FP/CAC teaching.

Overall, the goal was for faculty participants to be able to:

- understand the principles of CBE
- revise course syllabi
- examine effective ways of lecturing
- discuss the variety of teaching methods that can be employed in clinical training
- demonstrate clinical skills teaching in a simulated setting
- develop good exam items for knowledge assessment
- assess skills, particularly using objective structured clinical examination (OSCE)
- apply the new medical eligibility criteria for family planning
- apply new recommendations in abortion care delivery
- demonstrate insertion of postpartum IUDs

#### Introduced Simulation-Based Training

The project also focused on the role of simulation-based training in advancing skills in the provision of contraception and pregnancy termination. UM-CIRHT exposed faculty and the school leadership to a multitude of trainings in teaching clinical skills, including delivery of contraception and pregnancy termination, using simulation; such instruction had been limited at most medical schools in Ethiopia before this. While skills laboratory teaching was indicated in the original curricula, in reality, the quality and frequency with which they were utilized were low to nonexistent in some schools. There were multiple reasons for this, such as lack of availability of space, equipment, and time in the course schedule, as well as a need for technical skill support for faculty. UM-CIRHT trained faculty in the rationale for simulation-based teaching and in how to integrate it into the curriculum, use simulators to teach skills, and give feedback and assess student practice. UM-CIRHT supported the setup and renovation of simulation labs, as well as the training of simulation lab technicians to better facilitate skills teaching using equipment such as mannequins. Learning guides were also adapted to include skills in delivery of contraception and pregnancy termination, and standards were developed for effective clinical skills teaching, including tools for faculty self-assessment.

### Integrated Interactive Teaching Methods

Many of the faculty had never been trained in effective teaching skills, which is important to ensure information is presented in a manner conducive to learning. The UM-CIRHT education team therefore invested time in training faculty in teaching skills such as writing and facilitating case studies as well as those used in a clinical setting. Prior to the intervention, most classes were structured as didactic presentations, which is less engaging than other methods and does not accommodate multiple learning styles. In addition to the simulation-based training, other methods introduced included case-based learning and the flipped-classroom model. After participating in the training sessions, each school received at least two follow-up visits from the education team to monitor the translation of training into practice.

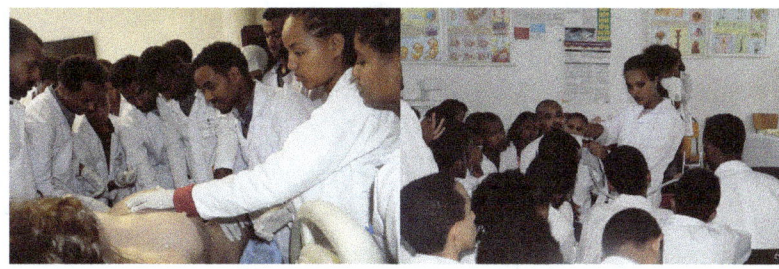

Simulation Lab Training at Addis Ababa University and Hawassa University

### Introduced Peer-Assisted Learning

Peer-assisted learning (PAL) is a form of academic support in which students mentor other students. The student mentors are trained in facilitation, coaching techniques, and general mentoring principles and meet regularly with mentees for study support sessions. The PAL scheme benefits students struggling with certain class content as well as the mentors by reinforcing course material and developing learning and creative skills. Mentors are undergraduate volunteers who have strong academic records and good communication skills. The education team introduced a pilot for PAL as a part of curriculum implementation at Addis Ababa University.

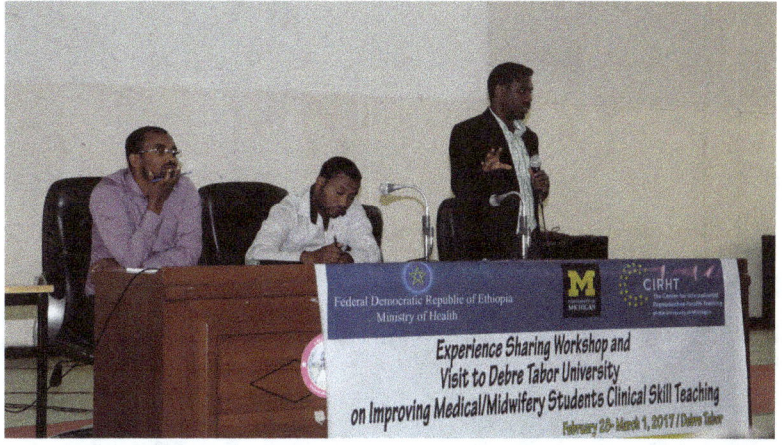

Workshop on Improving Clinical Skills Teaching at Debre Tabor University

*The Case of Bahir Dar University*

The OBGYN chair of Bahir Dar University highlighted the changes brought about by UM-CIRHT's partnership in teaching FP/CAC skills. In a presentation at the International Conference on Family Planning in November 2018, he recounted that the concept of simulation-based training was nascent in Ethiopian medical schools and that before the project there was no simulation center at his medical school. As a result of this project, the leadership at Bahir Dar dedicated space for a simulation center, renovating and equipping it with necessary FP/CAC simulators:

> *Of paramount importance was the focus on training faculty and senior residents on simulation-based training that included demonstrations, objective assessments, and debriefing. Sim center staff were equipped to handle mannequins and manage sim session scheduling. Apart from the infrastructure support, UM-CIRHT had spearheaded the development of guiding documents such as assessment tools, sim center guidelines, and skills logbooks, which faculty found eased and standardized skills teaching. With all of these inputs, medical students were trained on one skill per week in FP counseling, implant and IUD insertions and removals, and MVAs [manual vacuum aspirations]. Our school has now incorporated OSCE for the first time in its history, with two assessors at each sim station (one faculty and one senior resident). The OBGYN rotation now has formally incorporated OSCE assessment in all FP/CAC competencies. To date, 135 medical students have been objectively assessed in four rounds. We were encouraged by students' feedback: most had a positive experience with this relatively new assessment modality and recommended that it be continued in future evaluations. In sum, through simulation training, students are exposed to hands-on training [in] contraception and abortion skills.*

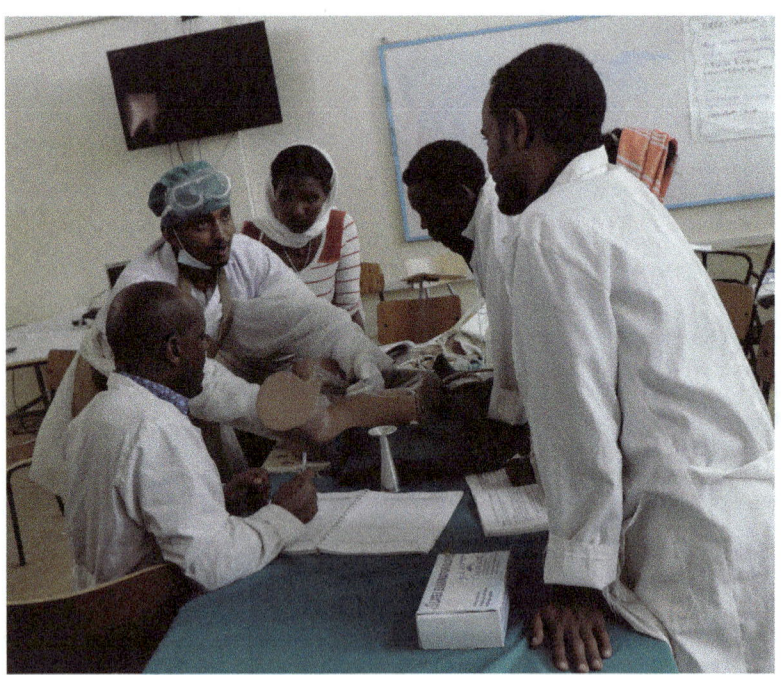

Simulation Lab at Bahir Dar University

### Assessment

*Standardized Student Logbooks*

As part of the effort to inculcate hands-on training in FP/CAC, the education team encouraged the use of standardized logbooks across the partner schools. For medical and midwifery students, they collaborated with the FMOH; for OBGYN residents, they worked with the Ethiopian Society of Obstetrics and Gynecology (ESOG). Students used their logbooks to record procedures they observed and/or performed during their FP clinical rotations. The logbooks were used for skills teaching, formed the basis of trainees' progressive assessments for FP/CAC, and were duly signed by supervising residents and/or attending physicians.

*Integrated New Learner Assessment Methods*

Aligning assessment methods with teaching objectives is a main component of CBE. The education team conducted multiple training sessions on appropriate assessment methods and tools and how to develop and apply the methods, including context-dependent multiple-choice examination and OSCE. OSCE testing is performance based and allows for the standardized assessment of a wide range of clinical skills. The education team members presented material on student assessment and worked with faculty to set up written and OSCE exams in real time. More than 75% of the faculty were subsequently trained in student assessment, and eight out of nine medical schools and six out of eight midwifery schools successfully introduced OSCE as an assessment method.

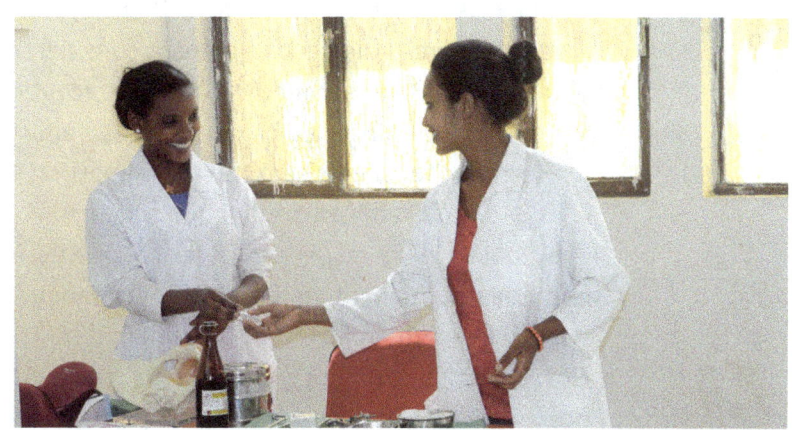

OSCE Assessment Preparation at Mekelle University

## Clinical Service Program

The ultimate goal of the project was to serve the needs of women and girls. That objective extended to clinical service at the teaching hospitals of the schools. It was important to provide FP/CAC in an easily accessible, woman-friendly, compassionate environment. The service program included not only the faculty, residents, and medical, nursing and midwifery students but also, in wider reach across hospitals and institutions, anyone who might interact with women and girls needing FP/CAC services. The teaching hospitals needed to have adequate caseloads to expose students to reproductive health (RH) service provision. Establishing high-quality RH services at these hospitals would have ripple effects on other health institutions, where these trained health cadres would be assigned after graduation. The main components of the clinical service program included:

- assessing the current FP/CAC service capacity
- establishing model clinics for FP/CAC service provision to enhance student rotation
- addressing abortion stigma through value clarification and attitude transformation (VCAT) training
- promoting the ethics and legal aspects of safe abortion
- developing educational materials for patients
- stimulating quality improvement committees and projects

### Assessed the Current FP/CAC Service Capacity

At the outset, the teaching hospitals affiliated with each partner school had different levels of service provision due to constraints on physical capacity, provider competence, or simple gaps in attention. Most hospitals offered FP services, but they were dispersed throughout the OBGYN wards as part of general service provisions. This meant the client population was not always aware of the availability of the services.

A team from UM-CIRHT worked with each school to provide a baseline assessment of the types of services offered and the facilities to support those services. Their first area of inquiry was determining whether there was available space for waiting, counseling, and procedures, as well as signage that clearly identified the availability of FP/CAC. They also considered basic sanitation needs like having a clean water supply, handwashing facilities, and toilets.

They also assessed the services themselves. This included looking at patient flow and medical records. The needs the team considered ran across the spectrum of FP: all temporary and permanent methods of contraception as well as first- and second-trimester abortions, including medical and surgical abortions. Their analysis also considered the waiting time for clients seeking a safe abortion in the first or second trimester.

The team examined staffing for specific FP services and which staff provided them. They looked at the respective roles of residents, interns, nurses, midwives, OBGYN faculty, and other permanent staff for FP/CAC. Among their questions were the following: What were the length and content of students' rotations through the clinics and procedures? How were those rotations logged and supervised? More broadly, the assessment looked at how services were being offered as a part of antenatal care, postpartum care, and general health care for women and girls.

Once the assessment was completed, the gaps were noted and a work plan was established jointly by representatives from the partner school and UM-CIRHT. This was used to promote changes such as the renovation of the physical environment, training to fill knowledge and practice gaps, and the introduction of new processes to monitor progress.

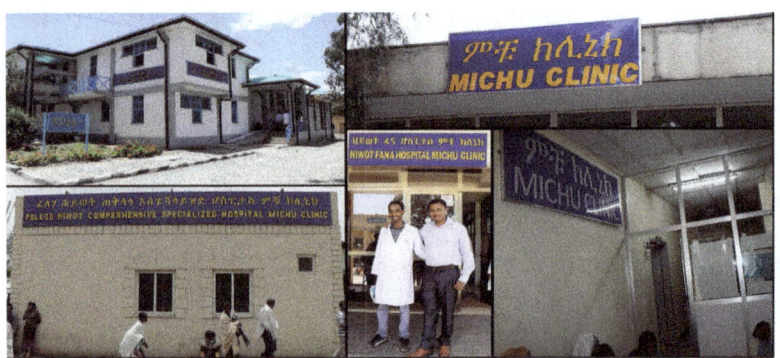

Michu Clinics, Clockwise from Top Left: Mekelle University, Addis Ababa University, Hawassa University, Haramaya University, and Bahir Dar University

### Established Model Clinics for FP/CAC Service Provision to Enhance Student Rotation

Based on the assessment, a plan was developed for model clinics that would serve as an extension of the classroom for students and provide exceptional FP/CAC care for women and girls. Such clinics were planned for each of the partner schools, branded *"Michu clinics,"* using an Amharic word meaning *"comfort"* to emphasize their welcoming culture. The build-out of these clinics involved renovation or construction at each of the partner schools to meet the standard of *"comfort"* aspired to for a Michu clinic. Sometimes a full clinic was established immediately and sometimes an interim facility was created while the designated rooms or areas awaited larger construction. The clinics had to have adequate waiting room areas, places for information about FP/CAC, and even television sets that could be used to broadcast educational videos. Requirements for the clinical practice areas were beds and basic medical implements, as well as more advanced equipment like ultrasound machines. Each clinic had to offer the full range of FP/CAC, including short-term methods of contraception (condoms and pills), long-acting reversible contraception (LARC; such as IUDs, implants and injections), permanent methods of contraception (bilateral tubal ligation), and medical and surgical methods for first- and second-trimester pregnancy termination. The services were offered for any OBGYN visit, with special attention to postabortion and postpartum FP. By the end of the project period, Michu clinics were established at each partner school.

### *Addressed Stigma of Abortion through VCAT Training*

Facilities and technical skills were not the only barriers to women accessing safe abortion and family planning care. Like many other countries, providers had to contend with the stress and stigma associated with the provision of these services, which some considered controversial, affecting their attitudes. VCAT workshops were conducted for providers (and in some cases, every worker who came into contact with patients, including guards and cleaning staff). These workshops ensured that providers had a thorough knowledge of their rights and responsibilities as health workers but also asked participants to think critically about their own values and prejudices regarding abortion care.

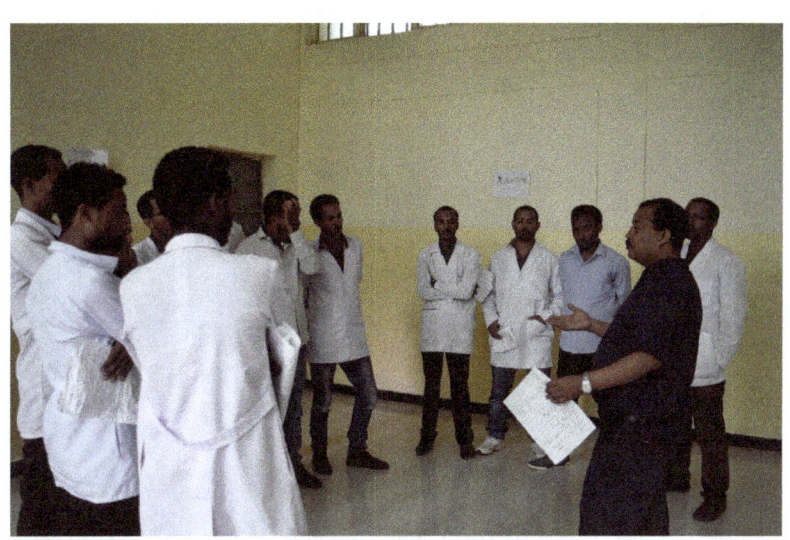

VCAT Training

### *Promoted Ethical and Legal Aspects of Safe Abortion*

After facilitating multiple VCAT workshops for various partner schools, the UM-CIRHT service team was unsatisfied with the overall response to the presentation of the material, which seemed to only have had a small effect on changing attitudes toward safe abortion.

They decided to shift the perspective of the content to ethics while keeping the overall aims of encouraging compassionate, patient-centered care and emphasizing reproductive justice. The revised presentation delved into providers' responsibilities to patients and society in general as advocates of policies that further the agenda of providing quality, evidence-based care to promote healthy lives for women.

### Promoted Patient Feedback and Education

For certain communications-related work, UM-CIRHT contracted with an outside vendor to understand the patient experience in the Michu clinics. The process began with handing out patient satisfaction surveys in the clinics to get feedback on what parts of the client experience were positive and what could be improved. The next steps were physical improvements, like developing recognizable branding and accessibility as well as redesigning clinical interiors and staff uniforms to be brighter and more pleasant. UM-CIRHT also contracted with another company to produce short educational videos in Amharic about implants and IUDs to be played in the waiting rooms of the Michu clinics.

### Stimulated Quality Improvement Committees and Projects

Quality improvement (QI) activities were deemed necessary to sustain developments in resident and student training and to continually stress aspects of service delivery, including patient satisfaction and adherence to contraception. The service team worked with each partner school to create QI committees, interdisciplinary groups of health care workers in FP/CAC that included OBGYN faculty, residents, midwives, and nurses. The QI committee at each partner school conducted a comprehensive baseline audit developed by UM-CIRHT to identify gaps in FP/CAC service quality. The audit consisted of 300 questions on process, patient care, outcome indicators, and other factors. The same audit was used at each location so monitoring would be consistent across sites. While each partner school audit produced different findings, there were some similarities across the schools: lack of availability of safe first-trimester abortion and PPFP services, long wait times for second-trimester abortion services, small or obscure FP clinic locations, and a lack of formal rotation in FP clinics for trainees.

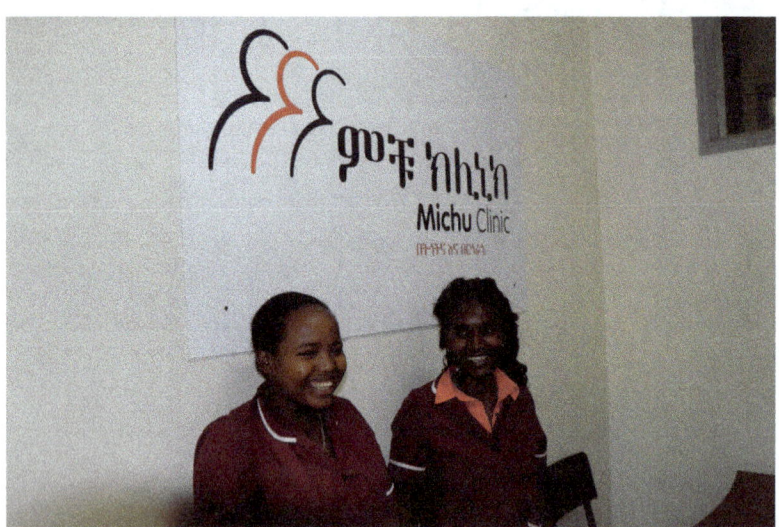

Michu Clinic at Hawassa University with New Uniforms and Signage

Once the gaps were identified, the service team organized and facilitated on-site workshops for each partner QI committee to review the baseline audit findings, prioritize gap areas, set goals, and develop intervention plans for QI project implementation. Some of the QI projects addressed in-service provider training in FP/CAC, assigning residents and interns to FP/CAC services, creating policy guidelines and standards of service, and renovating existing building space to establish an FP/CAC outpatient clinic. Using the PDCA (plan, do, check, act) cycle framework, the QI committees tested and assessed their interventions by adhering to data-collection routines, reviewing the collected data at bimonthly committee meetings, and working with the service team during regular supportive UM-CIRHT supervision visits.

Seminars and trainings focused on specific clinical issues as well as on patient-centered care with attention to counseling, communication, and patient satisfaction. Creating basic management tools like documentation practices and supply-chain management were also a part of the QI effort. QI committees at each site were responsible for implementing tools, identifying gaps in service provision, and creating QI projects to address those gaps.

### *The Case of Adama Hospital Medical College*

Each partner school experienced tangible results specific to its own context. In the case of Adama Hospital Medical College (AHMC), the Michu clinic was established with routine rotations for residents, interns, nurses, and midwives. The hospital dedicated nine beds specifically for second-trimester abortion, and PPFP saw a dramatic increase, rising to 30% uptake for women in the immediate postpartum phase. This was all accomplished despite significant challenges, including systemic problems like infrastructure issues, which influenced FP/CAC provision, and difficulties with money allocation when trying to distribute project funds, leading to delays in activities. Additional challenges faced at AHMC were a consistent shortage of staff, compounded by high staff turnover rates, which impacted service availability. Initial attempts at in-service training were stymied by per-diem and compensation issues.

Lessons learned from the QI experience at AHMC underscore the benefits of institutional QI projects, which can improve infrastructure and access to services, as well as the quality of care provided. This in turn can increase the number of clients, which increases opportunities for preservice training exposure.

One of the most important factors that helped AHMC achieve its success was the institutional and facility ownership of the project. A UM-CIRHT employee commented, *"The bold action of the college management, especially the provost, to hand over their offices to establish the*

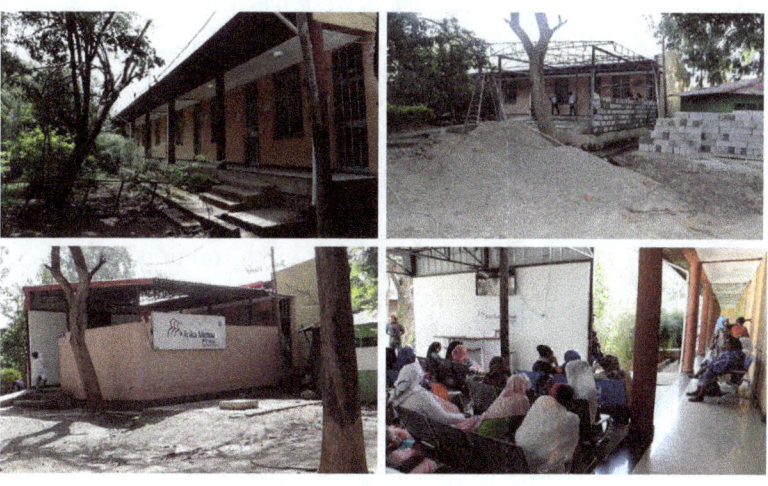

Renovation and Use of Adama's Michu Clinic

*Michu clinic in the hospital demonstrated an unprecedented commitment. This significantly minimized the prevailing space shortage for provision of RH services."* Not only did the staff and departments working in FP/CAC value the initiative, but the heads of the college and hospital did as well, which had a positive effect on access to these services. The process was another factor that led to AHMC's positive outcomes—by applying an evidence-based, participatory approach to QI, it was possible to increase service access and quality in a relatively short time span. Looking ahead, continued ownership and on-site support on all levels will be crucial to ensure the sustainability of these outcomes.

## Research Program

The research program aimed to strengthen and sustain a culture of research in FP/CAC and build faculty research capacity in partner health professional schools by providing optimal research skills through a systematic, longitudinal approach. To achieve this, UM-CIRHT supported tailored milestone-based research methodology training along the continuum of the research cycle, from the framing of a research question and data collection and analysis to manuscript writing and publication. Through this endeavor, the project aimed to increase the number of independent faculty investigators in the partner schools, which ultimately would lead to better evidence-based medical practice.

### *Conducted Baseline Assessment of Research Needs*

The research program began in early 2015 with a preliminary needs assessment of the then eight medical schools in Ethiopia. The baseline assessment revealed that OBGYN faculty lacked both protected time for research and dedicated research funding and had only limited knowledge and skills in conducting research. The faculty identified these as major factors contributing to the dearth of research activity and culture.

### *Built a Network of Research Advisors*

The research endeavor required creating a group of experienced research investigators who would be able to provide training, coaching, and peer feedback to faculty investigators at the partner schools. This included the members of the in-country and Michigan-based research team for UM-CIRHT, as well as others from their professional networks in Ethiopia and Michigan. The in-country advisors were able to easily travel to the partner schools to support research training. This in-country team was initially just the research director, who developed a scope of work and a road map for the implementation of the research program with the partner schools based on the findings of the baseline assessment. The team grew to include two research coordinators who provided on-site supportive supervision to the research teams at the partner schools during various stages of the research life cycle. The research coordinators facilitated the day-to-day work of the research teams at partner schools through the following activities:

- coordinating a series of on-site research methodology workshops taught by identified expert trainers within the partner schools, in-country, or through UM-CIRHT contacts
- providing periodic on-site supportive supervision for research project implementation
- serving as liaisons with other members of the UM-CIRHT research team
- advising on the budgets of the pilot research grants
- facilitating transfers of approved funds for the pilot research grants

### *Facilitated Inspirational Talks by Local Successful Researchers*

UM-CIRHT invited faculty at each respective school with a track record of conducting and publishing scholarly work in peer-reviewed journals to speak to junior faculty. These busy clinicians with established research careers spoke candidly to the faculty and delivered a series of talks on site in a workshop format. The inspirational talks were aimed at reinvigorating research, demystifying research conduct, and sharing practical tips, including time-management skills. Anecdotally, these talks have inspired other faculty who until then had only been peripherally exposed to research.

### *Awarded Pilot Research Grants to Local Faculty Investigators*

In June 2015, UM-CIRHT launched a pilot research grant program that was open to all OBGYN faculty at the partner schools. In February 2017, a second round of pilot research grants was opened to the midwifery faculty at the partner schools. Both followed an iterative, transparent process to award competitive pilot grants based on clearly stipulated selection criteria with scientific and public health merit. Teams had to be multidisciplinary, involving coinvestigators from other clinical departments or sciences. During the selection process, principal investigators (PIs) incorporated input from seasoned investigators across medical, midwifery, and public health schools and the FMOH. Once selected, UM-CIRHT paired the PIs with mentors from U-M who were experienced research investigators. These research projects were used as examples in hands-on activities throughout the faculty research workshops.

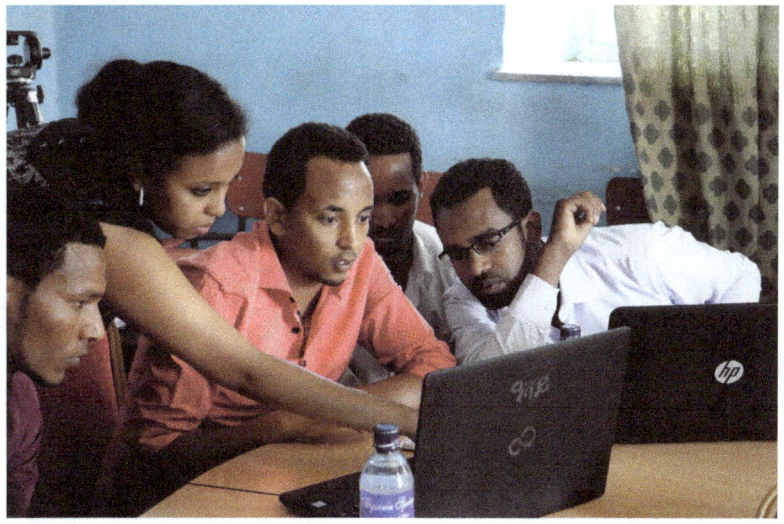

Research Training at the University of Gondar

*Facilitated Research Training and Coaching throughout the Research Life Cycle*

UM-CIRHT organized a series of research workshops to inspire a positive research culture and strengthen the capacity of local faculty. The workshops followed the full life cycle of a research project (see figure 6) with the aim of equipping junior faculty with the skills necessary to lead such a project from the initial selection of a research question through to the publication of the results in a scientific journal. All faculty in OBGYN and midwifery were able to attend, not just those faculties selected for the pilot research grants.

*Milestones in the Research Life Cycle*

Step 1. Frame the Research Question
At each site, experienced researchers led hands-on workshops in framing appropriate research questions. Through didactics and interaction sessions, participants discussed

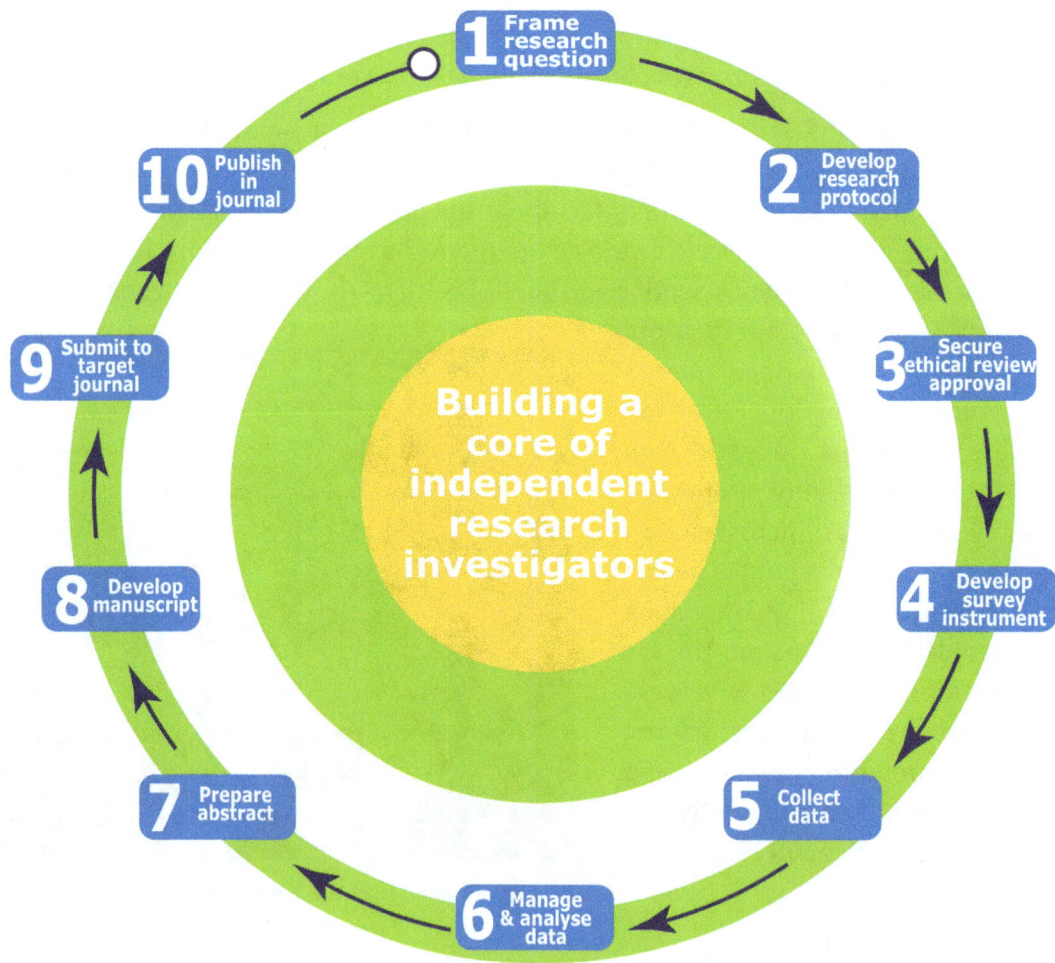

Figure 6. Research Milestones to Build a Cadre of Independent Investigators at Partner Schools

the importance of a well-defined research question(s) before moving to the next phases of conduct. Faculty—and, in some cases, residents too—formed teams and critiqued the merits of research questions through a priori–defined criteria. Specifically, trainers emphasized the FINER (feasible, interesting, novel, ethical, relevant) criteria of judging the merits of good research questions with adaptation to include that of the National Institutes of Health (NIH) for research grants (significance, approach, innovation). These exercises helped faculty develop and submit research questions of interest for potential funding and laid the groundwork for the selection process.

*Step 2. Develop the Research Protocol*
The objective of the research protocol workshop was to enable investigators to turn their research question into fully formed research proposals based on their specific aims. By the end of the workshop, faculty had developed draft proposal documents that had the major elements of research protocols, including research methods and data-analysis plans. As in the other research workshops, these sessions lasted four to five days and were highly interactive, structured with the workshop leader(s) functioning as facilitators. Participation was open to all faculty, including those who may not have had their research topics selected. Feedback from faculty, coinvestigators, and other research team members confirmed that the sessions had been valuable and, more important, useful.

Following the workshop, the research teams were given approximately one month to further revise and refine their research protocols. They were expected to interact with their team members, adapt their protocols, and seek advice on their research design and data-analysis plans with local biostatistics experts in their respective schools of public health. They also worked on their proposed budget plans.

Once those revisions were made, local defense sessions were held at each of the partner schools with the objective of strengthening the proposals to make them more competitive. Local public health or epidemiology faculty led the sessions and provided rankings against a set of preformed criteria, as well as giving constructive feedback on methodology. Each presentation lasted 20 minutes. Site coordinators facilitated the defenses with support from the UM-CIRHT research team. Scoring at local defense sessions determined which ones proceeded to the national research protocol defense. OBGYN and midwifery each had their own local and national defenses.

For the national defense, research proposals were presented over two days. The judges were experts in reproductive health and/or had methodological or statistical expertise and were selected from the faculty of universities across the country and experts from the FMOH Department of Maternal, Newborn, and Child Health. The judges scored each of the presentations using set criteria and also provided feedback on the protocols. One stakeholder from the FMOH commented, *"If there is a policy intent of the research, engaging the ministry in selection of topics can focus it more on monitoring and generating evidence that can be applied nationally."* The FMOH representatives provided a perspective to align the selected projects with topics of national interest and relevance. In fact, the FMOH input directly inspired the creation of two of the research projects.

The average scores from all the judges were summed up to rank the research projects. After the defense, the strongest projects were selected for pilot grant support from UM-CIRHT. The PIs were expected to revise the protocols based on input from the judges. The UM-CIRHT research team was in regular contact with the PIs via phone, email, and in-person meetings to ensure that the feedback was incorporated into their proposals. In parallel with these revisions, the research team evaluated the budget proposals of each of the selected projects against their justifications.

*Step 3. Secure Ethical Review Approval*
The PIs submitted their revised protocols to their respective institutional review boards (IRB) for ethical approval. This was an essential step to ensure adherence to human-subject research guidelines, and no funding was released without such ethical clearance.

*Step 4. Design the Survey Instrument*
Almost all the research projects selected for pilot grant support involved primary data collection (with a few retrospective chart reviews) and as such needed support through the development of research instruments. Even if the proposals submitted initially had some data-capturing elements, they may not have been well developed.

The survey instrument workshop helped the teams refine their tools. While this was an iterative process, the two- to three-day workshop led by local public health experts helped inculcate fundamental tool-development principles and practical hands-on skills in each of the teams. Quantitative and qualitative research tools were covered during these sessions, since some teams had both methods included in their projects. For two of the multicenter studies, besides the local workshop and individual mentors' input, the forum at the Program on Women's Healthcare Effectiveness Research (PWHER) group within the U-M OBGYN department provided substantial feedback on the survey instruments, as well as focus group and in-depth interview guides. These revised tools were used to help collect the primary data in an analyzable format. Once survey instruments were fully developed, teams converted them into appropriate data-collecting formats and translated the documents into local languages. While most used paper for collecting their data, a few teams had developed electronic data-capturing tools and were able to collect their data directly on tablets.

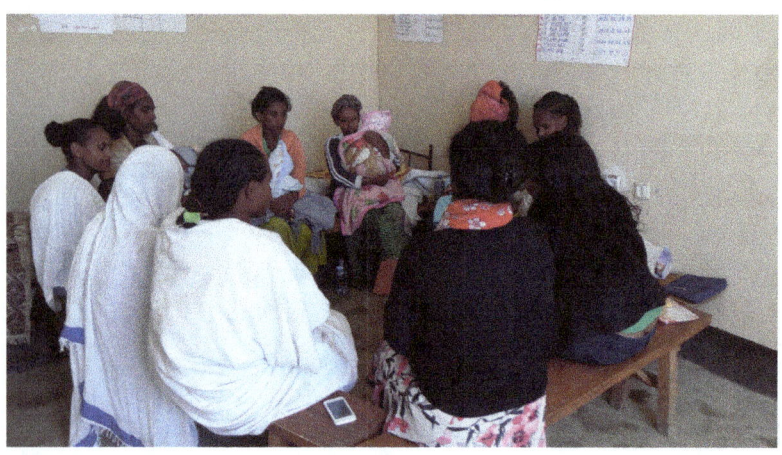

Data Collection in a Village near Mekelle

*Step 5. Collect the Data*
Research teams recruited data collectors and trained them on the projects and data-collection procedures. Recruitment and deployment of data collectors varied across the teams and schools. The UM-CIRHT research team and site coordinators served in supporting roles when teams came upon issues, such as difficulties determining benchmark payment rates for data collectors and identifying research coordinators.

*Step 6. Manage and Analyze Data*
Once the teams had reached their target sample size, they completed workshops in data management and analysis taught by statisticians versed in analytic frameworks—preferably public health experts and biostatisticians whenever possible. The workshops ran for three to five days, the duration dependent on the time the research team members were able to dedicate and the complexity of the analyses.

The objective of these workshops was to help teams clean up data and create analytic data files so they could run appropriate statistical analyses on their own. The workshops covered various types of data-analysis methods and when to use them, as well as commonly used statistical packages and quantitative-analysis software. By the end of the workshop, teams were each expected to have clean analytical data sets, an updated data-analysis plan, and preliminary inputs for the results section of their respective manuscripts.

*Step 7. Prepare Abstracts*
Authors created abstracts to summarize the research questions, methods, and resulting findings. The abstracts were later adapted to be proposals for research conferences or journal opportunities, depending on the scope.

UM-CIRHT identified relevant scientific conferences and encouraged PIs to prepare the abstracts and submit their scholarly work for presentation, creating a platform for interaction with global leaders in the field. With a priori–set criteria, faculty and residents were able to present their work in the form of oral and/or poster presentations at various national and international conferences in reproductive health.

*Step 8. Develop Manuscripts*
Research teams were encouraged to draft manuscripts structured according to a target journal they selected. Although the PIs were responsible for overseeing the manuscript drafting, all the coauthors were expected to intellectually contribute to the write-up in an iterative manner.

In many of the partner schools, faculty reported limited experience with developing full-length

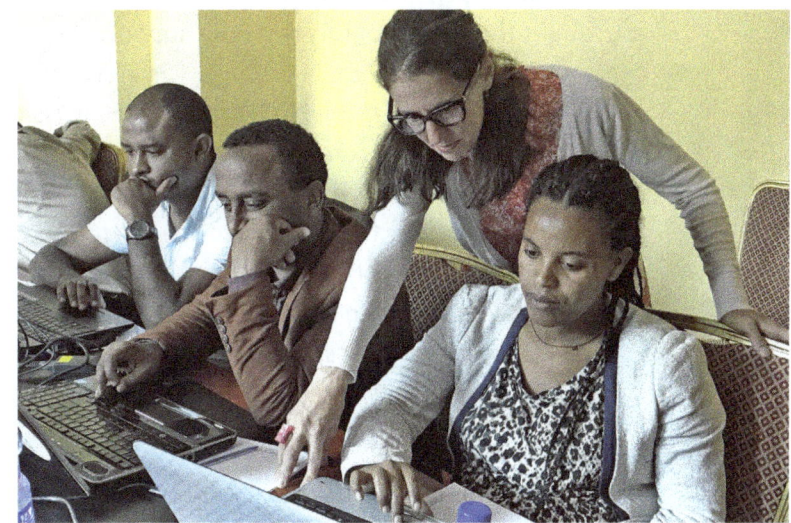
Scientific Writing Workshop

biomedical journal articles to submit to peer-reviewed journals. To support the research writing, UM-CIRHT partnered with U-M Pre-Publication Support Services (PREPSS), which has extensive experience supporting manuscript writing and publishing for authors from numerous low- and middle-income countries. This support included a four-day intensive hands-on writing workshop for all OBGYN PIs. PIs submitted their draft manuscripts prior to the on-site workshop to help gauge the training pace and common pitfalls that the authors were likely to encounter. By the end of the workshop, participants were expected to have a more refined manuscript and receive and respond to feedback from peer reviewers. As a follow-up to the workshop, PREPSS provided personalized manuscript development support to the PIs. The support included one-on-one consultations for peer-review and copyediting support.

*Step 9. Submit to Target Journal*
The PREPSS support included guidance on selecting a target journal and tailoring the manuscript to specific journal requirements, as well as templates for letters for corresponding with journal editors.

*Step 10. Publish in Journal*
As part of the research process, the UM-CIRHT team, PREPSS, and mentors stressed to PIs that the journal article process is often iterative—that the target journal may reject the paper and investigators will need to find alternative outlets. When a journal article is accepted from a journal, there are multiple rounds of feedback with the editor and reviewers for revisions to content and layout. PIs were coached through this process up to the point of final publication.

### The Case of Hawassa University

The research capacity–building efforts paid dividends early on, as evidenced by the excitement of faculty who were motivated to carry out further research and consider the physician-scientist track. An OBGYN faculty member at Hawassa University commented about the impact of this research support:

> *I have been on the OBGYN faculty at Hawassa for the last eight years. I have participated in several research methodology workshops while in training and service. However, the only research project I completed was my thesis requirement for residency. I did not get the opportunity to see the full breadth of [the] clinical research endeavor until [this project]. The custom-made phase-based approach was very enticing, motivating, and engaging. I was fortunate to be one of the awardees of the competitive [pilot] grants. It inspired me to get out of my shell and collaborate with experts in other disciplines, including the public health school. The research training equipped me with the skills I needed to craft a relevant OBGYN research project using our hospital population. The grant motivated me to dedicate time to work on primary data collection and analysis in a team-based approach. I was one of the first grantees to complete data collection.*

> **RESEARCH ARTICLE**          **Open Access**
>
>
>
> # Surgical informed consent in obstetric and gynecologic surgeries: experience from a comprehensive teaching hospital in Southern Ethiopia
>
> Million Teshome[1*], Zenebe Wolde[1], Abel Gedefaw[1], Mequanent Tariku[1] and Anteneh Asefa[2,3]
>
> ## Abstract
>
> **Background:** Surgical Informed Consent (SIC) has long been recognized as an important component of modern medicine. The ultimate goals of SIC are to improve clients' understanding of the intended procedure, increase client satisfaction, maintain trust between clients and health providers, and ultimately minimize litigation issues related to surgical procedures. The purpose of the current study is to assess the comprehensiveness of the SIC process for women undergoing obstetric and gynecologic surgeries.
>
> **Methods:** A hospital-based cross-sectional study was undertaken at Hawassa University Comprehensive Specialized Hospital (HUCSH) in November and December, 2016. A total of 230 women who underwent obstetric and/or gynecologic surgeries were interviewed immediately after their hospital discharge to assess their experience of the SIC process. Thirteen components of SIC were used based on international recommendations, including the Royal College of Surgeon's standards of informed consent practices for surgical procedures. Descriptive summaries are presented in tables and figures.
>
> **Results:** Forty percent of respondents were aged between 25 and 29 years. Nearly a quarter (22.6%) had no formal education. More than half (54.3%) of respondents had undergone an emergency surgical procedure. Only 18.4% of respondents reported that the surgeon performing the operation had offered SIC, while 36.6% of respondents could not recall who had offered SIC. All except one respondent provided written consent to undergo a surgical procedure. However, 8.3% of respondents received SIC service while already on the operation table for their procedure. Only 73.9% of respondents were informed about the availability (or lack thereof) of alternative treatment options. Additionally, a majority of respondents were not informed about the type of anesthesia to be used (88.3%) and related complications (87.4%). Only 54.2% of respondents reported that they had been offered at least six of the 13 SIC components used by the investigators.
>
> **Conclusions:** There is gap in the provision of comprehensive and standardized pre-operative counseling for obstetric and gynecologic surgeries in the study hospital. This has a detrimental effect on the overall quality of care clients receive, specifically in terms of client expectations and information needs.
>
> **Keywords:** Surgical informed consent, Obstetrics and gynecology, Clients, Counseling

Journal Article Published by Research Investigator at Hawassa University

Journal article cover page used under a Creative Commons Attribution 4.0 International License.

This faculty member was the first PI to publish his work in a peer-reviewed journal.[8] After that accomplishment, this investigator started a follow-up research project and applied for an internal grant for Hawassa University faculty.

## Faculty Development Program

The faculty development program provided faculty in the OBGYN, midwifery, nursing, and collaborating departments with the skills, coaching, and professional networks to effectively meet the education, service, and research program goals. The faculty development program drew upon a network of in-country experts as well as UM-CIRHT, U-M faculty and staff, and connections at other universities, and it covered targeted training interwoven with the other three program areas—education, service, and research—as well as the crosscutting topics that spanned all three. Activities included the following:

- conducting workshops for education, service, and research objectives
- stimulating leadership coaching to develop institutional change agents
- brokering experience-sharing visits between peer institutions
- contributing to global dialogue at renowned RH academic conferences
- convening video conferences to connect U-M mentors with partner school faculties

### *Conducted Targeted Workshops for Education, Service, and Research Objectives*

As mentioned in the earlier sections, each of the program areas included workshops and coaching for faculty. For the education program, these workshops focused on curriculum review and design, CBE, OSCE, simulation-based training, and exam blueprint preparation and item development. For the service program, topics included various short-acting, long-acting, and permanent methods of contraception; medical and surgical abortion for first- and second-trimester pregnancies; VCAT; ethical and legal aspects of abortion; client-centered counseling; and compassionate and respectful care. For the research program, workshop topics included information literacy, data analysis, and writing. A full list of topics is provided in figure 15.

### *Stimulated Leadership Coaching to Develop Institutional Change Agents*

The culture change goals envisioned at the partner schools required strong change management. Almost all leaders at the helm of the OBGYN and midwifery and nursing departments agreed on the relevance of the project and their schools' goals. However, the implementation required that the entire school's leadership be brought on board and exposed to training on how to become a change agent. Core faculty at all levels of educational leadership from the partner schools received training and continuous remote mentoring. The leadership training included workshops and team and individualized coaching. UM-CIRHT partnered with an Ethiopian company to facilitate the process, which was intended to help faculty in leadership positions initiate and sustain change within their institution—and within themselves. Faculty were given tools to overcome institutional and individual resistance and introduce initiatives for improving academia overall. Workshop participants came up with project ideas that they committed to lead in their respective departments, including improving teaching, transforming the work climate, and setting standards for clinical service. Each partner school created four to five groups, each made up of several individuals.

### *Brokered Experience-Sharing Visits between Peer Institutions*

Once embarking on these change-management goals in FP/CAC at their institutions, it was valuable for the partner school faculty to connect with peers who had completed similar projects at other institutions. Faculty completed experience-sharing visits for multidirectional knowledge exchange within and between countries. Faculty described these opportunities as *"precious"* for their own professional development. These visits included the following:

- a trip by the faculty champions to the University of British Columbia's Women's Hospital and Comprehensive Abortion and Reproductive Education (CARE) Program Women's Health Centre
- a multischool educational workshop at Debre Tabor University that included 45 participants across the partner schools
- a visit focused on PPFP hosted by Adama Hospital Medical College for providers from Bahir Dar University and Mekelle University
- an attachment for OBGYN residents and midwifery students at University of Mekelle with affiliate hospitals

### *Contributed to Global Dialogue at Renowned RH Academic Conferences*

The goal of the research program was to generate evidence to improve education, service, and knowledge about FP/CAC. In order to enhance that research, UM-CIRHT coached and supported faculty at national and international academic conferences. This included participating in renowned conferences focused on RH and in increasing RH imprint at other mainstream health conferences. Through its website, blog, and social media, UM-CIRHT promoted the partner schools' presence at these events, which helped make the faculty work more visible. These conferences included the following:

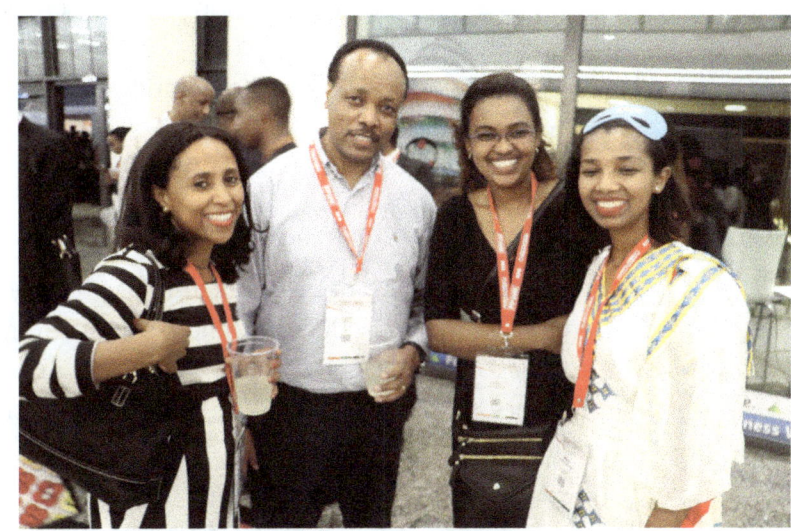

Ethiopian colleagues attending the International Conference on Family Planning in Kigali, Rwanda, November 2018

- October 2015—21st World Congress of Gynecology and Obstetrics organized by the International Federation of Gynecology and Obstetrics (FIGO) in Vancouver, Canada
- January 2016—4th International Conference on Family Planning (ICFP) in Nusa Dua, Indonesia
- January 2016—3rd International Congress on Women's Health and Unsafe Abortion (IWAC) in Bangkok, Thailand
- May 2016—4th global conference of Women Deliver in Copenhagen, Denmark
- November–December 2016—Africa Regional Conference on Abortion in Addis Ababa, Ethiopia
- March 2017—6th annual conference of Ethiopia Public Health Officers Association (PHOA-E) in Addis Ababa, Ethiopia

- April 2017—53rd Annual Medical Conference of the Ethiopian Medical Association (EMA) in Addis Ababa, Ethiopia
- April 2017—five-kilometer walk/run celebrating the theme *"Family Planning for Prosperity"* sponsored by the Ethiopian Medical Association (EMA) in Addis Ababa, Ethiopia
- May 2017—25th annual celebration of the Ethiopian Midwives Association (EMWA) in Addis Ababa, Ethiopia
- June 2017—31st congress of the International Confederation of Midwives (ICM) in Toronto, Canada
- March 2018—9th Annual Consortium of Universities for Global Health (CUGH) Conference in New York, US
- May 2018—26th International Day of the Midwife conference organized by the Ethiopian Midwives Association (EMWA) in Addis Ababa, Ethiopia
- October 2018—22nd World Congress of Gynecology and Obstetrics organized by the International Federation of Gynecology and Obstetrics (FIGO) in Rio de Janeiro, Brazil
- November 2018—5th International Conference on Family Planning (ICFP) in Kigali, Rwanda

### Convened Video Conferences to Connect U-M Mentors with Partner School Faculty

Video conferencing was a useful interface for webinars, online meetings, and journal club group discussions with faculty and residents from the partner schools. Journal club topics included contraception, safe abortion, new developments in RH research and care, and evidence-based medicine (EBM). EBM involves the careful and systematic application of rules of evidence to a study to assess its validity, importance, and usefulness in clinical practice and decision-making. Prior to the webinar and journal club sessions, participants were assigned papers and specific sections to read and critique in advance. During the discussion, each presenter walked the participants through the selected paper and analyzed each aspect of the study in an interactive manner.

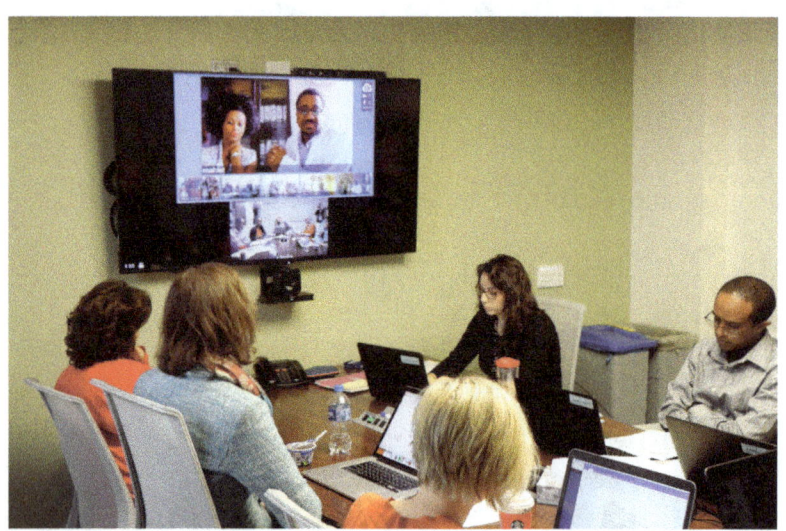

Journal Club, Started at the University of Michigan with Participants from Six Ethiopian Campuses

### Monitoring and Evaluation

The monitoring and evaluation (M&E) activities were designed to align project implementation with the intended outcomes in preservice medical and midwifery training. M&E data were collected regularly on project activities to determine whether progress was being made as planned, to gather feedback, and to suggest and implement any necessary corrective actions. The M&E framework used a log frame approach for collecting information pertaining to the implementation of its activities. The *log frame* is a matrix of activities developed from the project's outset in consultation with stakeholders at partner institutions. It details the logical steps in implementing the program, including inputs, processes, outputs, outcomes, and impact (see figure 7).

The target outcomes of the project included improved adherence to the harmonized and integrated curriculum, simulation lab usage and hands-on training, stronger competency in FP/CAC among new graduates, and greater involvement of faculty in FP/CAC-service delivery and teaching. The project also aimed to see increases in graduate and faculty research and its rigor, the number of RH publications, and participants' competitiveness for external grant-funding opportunities.

The M&E approach was developed in collaboration with faculty champions and site coordinators from the partner schools. This open process promoted stakeholder buy-in, aligned planned activities and investments with expected results, set performance indicators, and designated responsibilities across the team. Through this approach, the project goals were verified with the M&E team and aligned with the higher-level strategies of the partner schools.

### *Standardized Data Collection*

The M&E team developed templates to standardize data collection across all the partner schools. Templates were created for each program area and were originally developed as documents or spreadsheets, though they were later adapted into an online database.

In the area of education, data were gathered every six months. Indicators included the following:

- frequency of FP/CAC core syllabus use for OBGYN and midwifery
- number of teaching hours for didactics and simulation in FP/CAC
- number of hours and procedures in the Michu clinic
- learner outcomes in written, OSCE, and other assessments

Prior to graduation, students completed a pregraduation assessment that tested for competencies in FP/CAC services.

In the area of clinical services, data were collected monthly by the site coordinator. Custom data-collection forms were created to expand upon the national RH indicators already required by the FMOH on paper and through its electronic health management information system (HMIS). Indicators related to clinical services included the following:

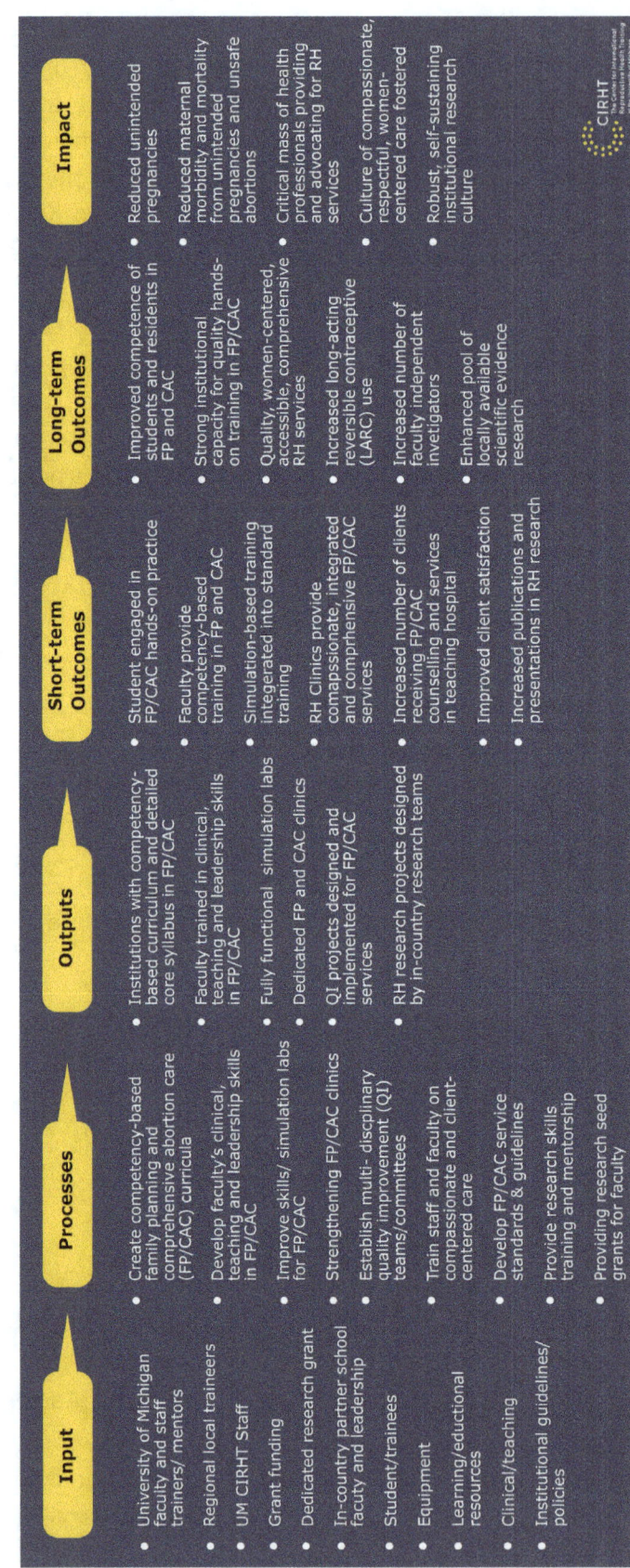

Figure 7. M&E Approach of UM-CIRHT Framework

- number of patients who had received FP/CAC services by which method
- number of deliveries
- PPFP uptake
- number of patients who received safe abortion or postabortion care
- postabortion family planning (PAFP) uptake

In the area of research, data were collected every two to three months. A short form was developed to track the status of each of the research projects. The template captured the progress in the research cycle, related funding, publications, and conferences.

The M&E team conducted periodic data audits to validate the data reported in the forms. For the service data, this included comparing the forms against the written service logbooks and electronic health record systems. In some cases, one-on-one follow-up with faculty was required for the research and education data.

### *Provided On-Site Quarterly Supervision*

A representative from the M&E team made a quarterly site visit to each partner school. During the site visit, they met with the faculty champions, site coordinators, and other leaders to make sure the agreed-on activities were proceeding as planned, to acknowledge good practices, to identify challenges and discuss possible solutions, and to listen to feedback for improvement in coordination with UM-CIRHT and internal coordination within the partner school. In between visits, the M&E team did routine follow-up via email with the site coordinators at each of the partner schools.

### *Conducted Stakeholder Interviews*

In October 2017, two members of UM-CIRHT conducted an assessment visit to the partner schools. Over a three-week visit, the team interviewed 95 individuals. The stakeholders approached for the final evaluation were leaders of the college or university in roles such as provost, dean, vice president, chief executive director (CED), chief academic and research director (CARD), and department head of OBGYN, nursing, or midwifery schools, as well as faculty in these departments who acted as former or current faculty champions for the project. Of those interviewed, 43% were in a leadership role and 57% in a faculty role. Of respondents, 72% (68 interviewees) were from medical school leadership or OBGYN departments and 28% (27 interviewees) from midwifery school leadership or faculty.

## Transition

At the start of phase 3 in August 2018, oversight of the project transitioned to the Ethiopian FMOH. The scope of phase 3 was determined mostly by the FMOH national priorities for FP/CAC and was moderately influenced by the results of the 2017 stakeholder interviews. The project transition activities were integrated into the annual FMOH planning process. The main objective of the transition work was to continue the shared priority of building the capacity of OBGYN and midwifery faculty in FP/CAC teaching and research. Seven of the former UM-CIRHT project staff based in Addis Ababa were *"seconded"* to the FMOH—that is, funded through external sources but reporting to FMOH directors. The seconded staff joined the FMOH as technical advisors within several directorates, including human resources development and quality improvement, and continued the coordination with the nine partner schools. The staff was oriented on the overall objectives and key activities of the directorates in which they embedded. The team was tasked with bridging the FP/CAC activities introduced through the project with routine delivery of RH curriculum and services at their schools and continued alignment with the national priorities of the health sector.

The FMOH saw the UM-CIRHT project as aligned with its own goals. In an April 2018 letter to the UM-CIRHT managing director, then Minister of Health Yifru Berhan Mitke wrote,

> *We believe that we cannot succeed in achieving our nationally set goals without meaningful empowerment of women and girls as tangibly expressed in the form of fighting and removing the prevailing barriers to decide in their own reproductive health. . . . The preservice training approach of UM-CIRHT to address the subject of reproductive health has been able to target medical students, OBGYN residents and midwives who after graduation would fan out into all parts of the country to offer quality and [the] full spectrum of reproductive health services in a dignified, caring, respectful and compassionate fashion. This implementation method of UM-CIRHT is not only cost-effective and results-oriented, it also ensures country ownership and sustainability.*

The incorporation of UM-CIRHT's activities into the overall work of the FMOH was another step toward sustaining progress in FP/CAC training and service delivery.

## Outcomes

### Overall

The FMOH was a constant partner, and the project reflected its overall strategy for improving health outcomes across the country in every discipline. The focus on specific institutions and on FP/CAC were elements that fit into the FMOH's own strategic planning and implementation.

Strong institutional ownership with shared goals and good communication was found to be crucial for adherence to educational changes and overall sustainability. Similarly, communication and coordination across partner schools were important for planning the curriculum changes. Flexibility was key when planning faculty development. Fostering trusting and respectful relationships with educators is important, and working with faculty to create schedules that were conducive with their other responsibilities was a large part of that.

All stakeholders agreed on the crucial role played by the site coordinators. Employed by UM-CIRHT but based at their respective sites, they were the nexus between the partner schools and the UM-CIRHT project office in Addis Ababa. They were educated and experienced in clinical care, and this understanding of the context and everyday challenges of the faculty working on the project allowed them to support faculty and staff on the ground. One of the largest challenges of implementing the project with UM-CIRHT was the lack of time available to faculty for new/additional responsibilities. Having someone on site who was dedicated to the project full time meant that data collection, monthly reports, and other tasks did not fall through the cracks. Many site coordinators took on other responsibilities such as facilitation of trainings and workshops and, at times, even patient care / clinical education at the Michu clinics.

One factor that admittedly may be difficult to duplicate elsewhere were preestablished social networks. Many people knew each other from previous professional or personal interactions, which meant that trust and communication were already established between many stakeholders. Department heads have the final say in scheduling, and without their approval, it is difficult to get resident or faculty time. Therefore, these personal relationships with management were very helpful. More generally, the energy and enthusiasm of the partner schools, stemming from the clarity of the shared goals and strategy, made it easier for different stakeholders to work together. Partnering faculty were allowed space to identify problems and challenges, and plans were then made to address these specific situations. Because of this equitable approach to partnering, UM-CIRHT gained a generally positive reputation, making new and potential partners eager to join the project. Internal staffing was another important component, with specialized teams and little turnover through the end of phase 2, allowing for consistency in on-the-job mentoring and other forms of technical support.

Addressing the stigma associated with CAC within the partner schools required a lot of outreach. During the initial rollout of VCAT training, UM-CIRHT's QI team noticed that participants were overwhelmingly opposed to the approach. The transition from VCAT to ethics- and law-focused training was a direct response to this realization and was received much more positively. Additionally, in line with the aforementioned importance of institutional buy-in, the general approach and attitude of leadership (e.g., provosts, department heads) was followed by residents and faculty with regard to CAC. If school leadership supported FP/CAC, the project implementation would run smoothly. If not, then residents and faculty would resist implementation.

From the outset of the project, M&E was an integral part of implementation. Consistent data over time would allow a deeper understanding of which interventions were working and which were not and why that might be the case. The M&E team worked closely with the site coordinators and the partner schools to be sure data were collected methodically, consistently, and accurately. While there were some changes made to the overall M&E framework during the project period, including in indicators and templates, the data amassed showed that the interventions yielded positive results. The M&E framework will continue to evolve, but the consistency of the data collection is something UM-CIRHT will continue to prioritize.

Another lesson was the necessity of strong project management to ensure that the objectives are met regarding the scope, budget, and timeline. With such a large network of individuals and organizations and the ambitious scope, project management admittedly varied, taking a more agile and adaptive approach rather than a tightly controlled, prescriptive one. This meant that priority activities were achieved successfully, but some lower-priority activities were done sparingly. Ensuring that all stakeholders were able to communicate was especially challenging. As the project and team grew from phase 1 to phase 2, some interviewees noted a lack of cohesiveness across programs within UM-CIRHT. With multiple organizations and turnover within the partner schools, some noted a lack of awareness about the high-level goals and responsibilities as specified in the MOU and that colleagues within the partner schools were not aware of the full range of resources available to them through the project: journals, equipment, coaching, and so on. Though many of the project objectives were met successfully, stronger internal project management and communication would have made the implementation much more efficient and effective.

Medical school leadership acknowledged the project as being timely and fortuitous, as it was well suited to their existing strategic goals of strengthening and expanding their medical education, research, and service portfolios. The leadership applauded UM-CIRHT's collaborative approach with their schools/departments and agreed that the project had exceeded their expectations in meeting the objectives set forth in the signed MOU. One leader stated that the *"[project] efforts thus far have benefited not only the departments of OBGYN and midwifery but have positively impacted other [units]."* The most visible spillover effects came from expanding the skills lab, establishing the Michu clinics, and training in research support.

## Education

By the end of phase 2, the medical student, midwifery student, and OBGYN resident curricula had been revised and put in place with a competency-based education approach in the areas specific to FP/CAC. Faculty were aware of the syllabi and the availability of supporting materials. Faculty from all schools had been trained in producing interactive e-learning materials for flipped-classroom formats and had created 10 video lectures on FP/CAC. An offline technology platform had been set up at all schools so that students could access e-learning materials on FP/CAC and other topics without requiring internet connectivity. Approximately 70 student leaders were trained on how to coach their peers in taking responsibility for their learning through the PAL program. Both mentors and mentees reported positive experiences in strengthening their knowledge of course subject matter and adjusting to university life.

By July 2018, all nine partner schools were using the revised curricula. The schools also had simulation labs that were actively used in teaching skills in FP/CAC. Most of the schools—eight of the nine medical schools and six of the eight midwifery schools—had introduced OSCE to assess skills in the provision of contraception and pregnancy termination. The institutions that had OSCE included at least one skill for FP and one for CAC.

Figure 8 shows OBGYN residents and medical and midwifery students across all nine partner schools by year of graduation. Figure 9 shows the number of students who completed written, oral and OSCE assessments between February 2017 and June 2018.

CBE became an objective way to apply learning objectives, delivered through simulation and multiple assessment methods to test skills and knowledge. The introduction of CBE in the areas of FP/CAC was found to have a broader impact on the institution, beyond just the OBGYN, nursing, and midwifery departments. In many instances, the CBE efforts lead to strengthened or increased institutional demand for an active, central health sciences education unit.

Effective coordination with national stakeholders was paramount for achieving a standardized curriculum and core syllabi across the nine partner schools. Those engaged included the FMOH and the FMOE as well as professional associations, specifically the

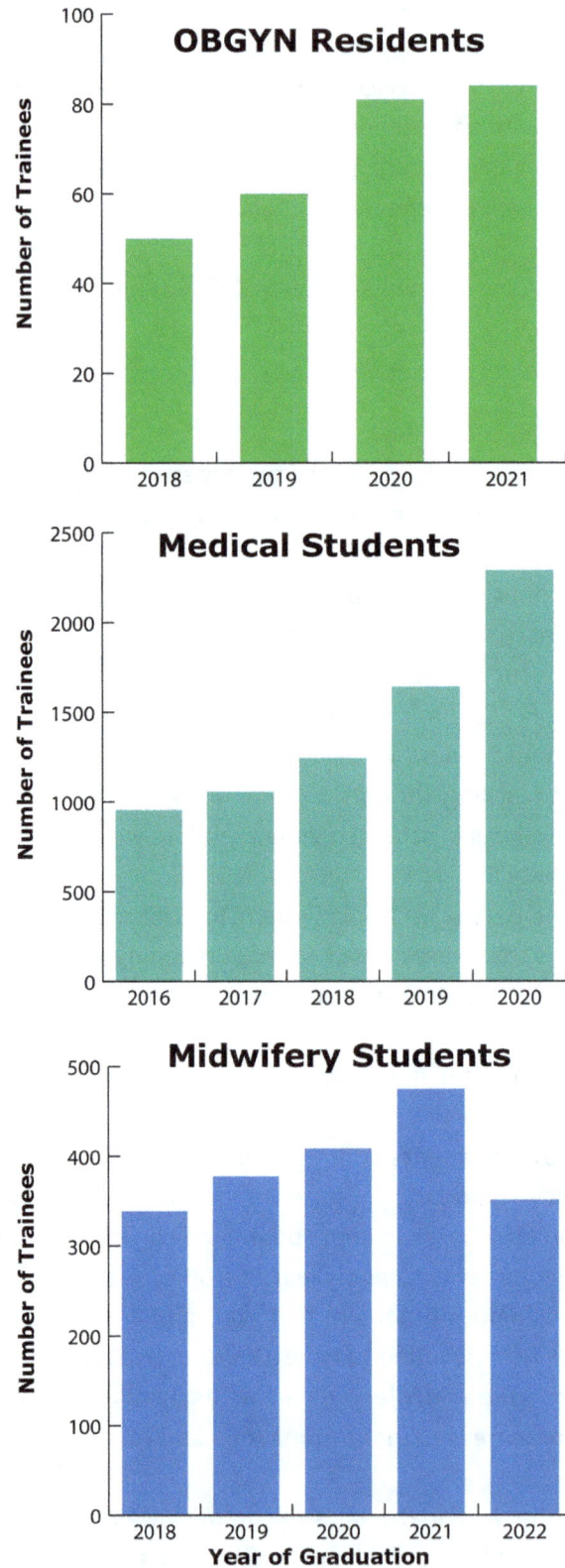

**Figure 8.** Student and Resident Enrollment across Partner Schools by Graduation Year

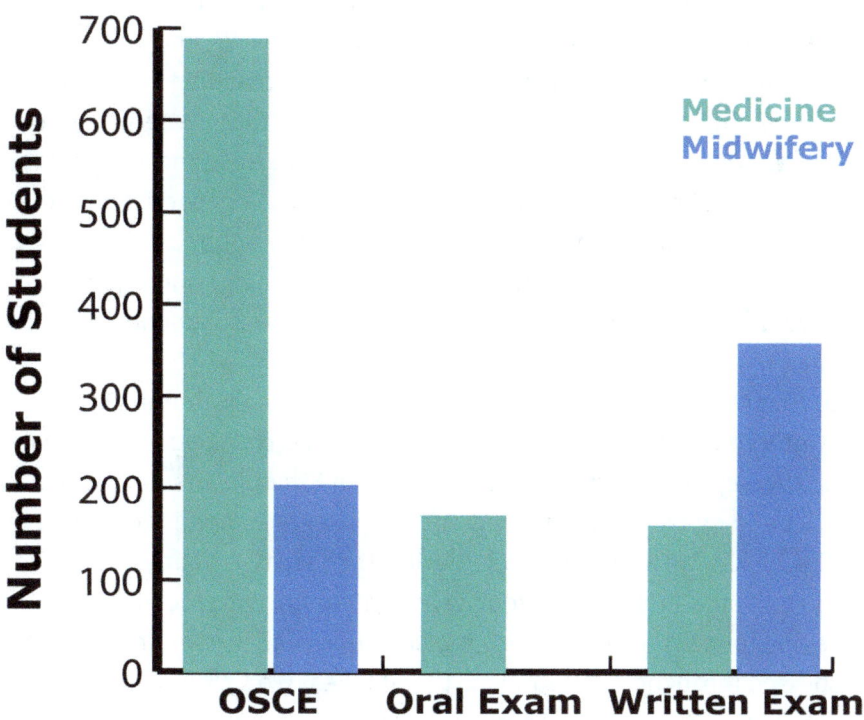

Figure 9. FP/CAC Assessments Conducted across Partner Schools, February 2017–June 2018

EMA, the EMWA, and the ESOG. By including these organizations in the project since phase 1, the partner schools were able to align their curriculum with national standards and priorities. This makes the curriculum changes more likely to continue after the project's end and also serves as a model for other public health sciences schools in Ethiopia looking to adopt a similar approach for including FP/CAC in preservice training.

Curriculum integration required rigorous and consistent follow-up through M&E as well as mentoring. This ensured that the revised curricula and content of faculty development training were translated into practice. The curricula revision and implementation process was a steep learning curve for many course instructors. Many of the faculty had no formal training on how to teach adults effectively and were used to didactic lectures as the sole means of instruction. Introducing new formats like case-based learning and simulation training required significant time and effort from course educators, many of whom had neither. Midwifery faculty faced additional difficulties, as most faculty were not clinical staff, and so there was a disconnect between classroom and clinical instruction. Some of the education challenges faced by partner schools were anticipated, as they are common challenges faced in many low-resource settings, such as low faculty-to-student ratio and high faculty turnover.

In the same vein, for implementation of simulation-based education, faculty and school leadership needed to provide consistent support. The integration of simulation-based teaching required leadership to allocate sufficient space for skills development centers, to continuously avail consumables, to replace and maintain mannequins and other equipment, and to assign technical staff for the center. It also took significant effort to encourage faculty to appreciate the importance of clinical skills teaching and assessment in a simulation setting. In phase 2, the project team observed that some simulation centers were not large enough to accommodate the large class sizes, and the low faculty-to-student ratio made it difficult for students to have adequate supervised practice on the simulation equipment. The stakeholders from the partner schools also expressed that training in simulation center management (such as scheduling) and equipment use and maintenance would be a valuable complement to promote the sustainability of simulation-based teaching.

Preservice training inherently takes a long-term approach to human resources development. One interviewee commented, *"Building capacity is changing culture, changing attitude, changing the way of doing things. It takes time."* In Ethiopia, medical school is four to seven years, depending on the curriculum and prior degrees, and is then followed by an internship. The FP/CAC intervention was during the last two years and the internship year. For midwifery students, it was a four-year curriculum, with the FP/CAC intervention in years three and four. OBGYN residency is also a four-year curriculum, with the FP/CAC topics interspersed throughout. This means that it takes two to four years for a student to complete the full FP/CAC training for his or her respective level. To date, there has not yet been a postdeployment survey of students who completed the full training. Therefore, the partner schools, the FMOH, and UM-CIRHT have not yet seen the impact of the preservice education intervention once graduates enter full-time practice as physicians and midwives.

For PAL implementation at Addis Ababa University, it was challenging to recruit and incentivize student volunteer mentors; social media was an effective tactic to recruit them. Both mentors and mentees reported positive experiences in strengthening knowledge on course subject matter and adjusting to university life.

### Clinical Service

By the end of 2018, all nine partner schools had operational Michu clinics. All the clinics provided comprehensive FP and safe abortion services led by OBGYN residents and supervised by nurses and OBGYN faculty. Preservice, students completed clinical rotations at the Michu clinics to experience FP/CAC service provision.

The Michu clinics had a dramatic effect on the availability, uptake, and quality of FP/CAC services. FP/CAC service utilization increased substantially; in many cases, it more than doubled. The number of faculty supportive of FP/CAC services increased dramatically due to UM-CIRHT's intervention. In the labor wards, PPFP was provided routinely across all partner schools. By the end of the implementation phase, all sites had established QI committees. The QI committees guided projects to continuously improve FP/CAC. Several of these projects were connected with research projects and developed into manuscripts or conference presentations.

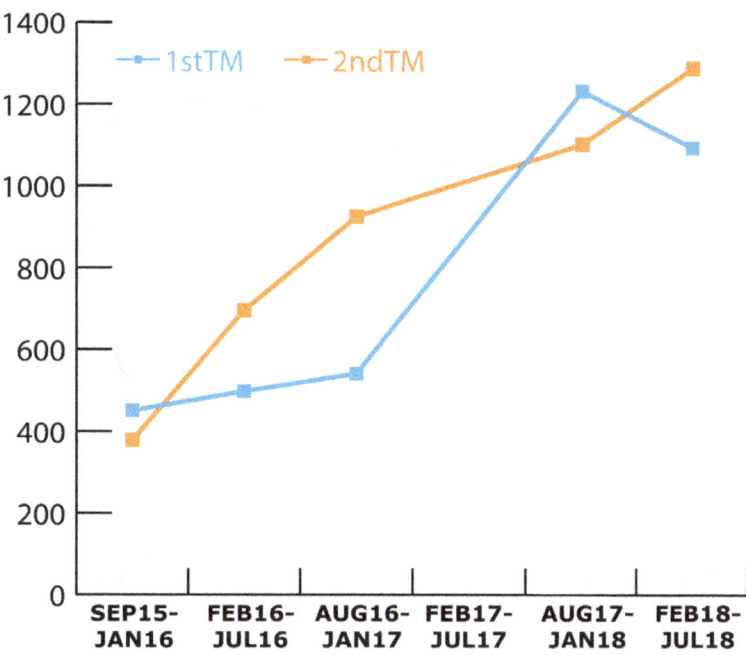

**Figure 10.** Safe Abortion Services by Trimester across Partner Schools, September 2015–July 2018

Figures 10–13 show the clinical service data, aggregated across partner schools in six-month intervals where complete data were available. Figure 10 shows the totals for safe abortions between September 2015 and July 2018, by trimester. Totals for both trimesters increased significantly, with second-trimester safe abortions increasing threefold over the nearly three-year time span.

Figure 11 shows total LARC use in relation to total FP services provided between September 2015 and July 2018. Both LARC and total FP show an upward trend (corresponding to the left y-axis). Importantly, the dotted line shows LARC as a percentage of FP (corresponding to the right y-axis), which also increases over time, indicating the increasing proportion of LARC usage among the FP user population. Figure 12 depicts PPFP in relation to total deliveries, between August 2016 and July 2018. While there is a large gap between the trend lines for total deliveries and PPFP (corresponding to the left y-axis), it is notable that the percentage of PPFP out of total deliveries (dotted line, corresponding to the right y-axis) increases steadily, from less than 6% to over 10% by July 2018.

Since these service data are aggregated across partner clinical sites, they do not convey the specific patterns by site or time interval.

Figure 13 shows PAFP in relation to total CAC services for the period between August 2016 and July 2018. Overall, an increase in both CAC and PAFP over time is observed. Additionally, there is an upward trend in the proportion of FP use following an abortion service by clients as depicted by the dotted line (right y-axis).

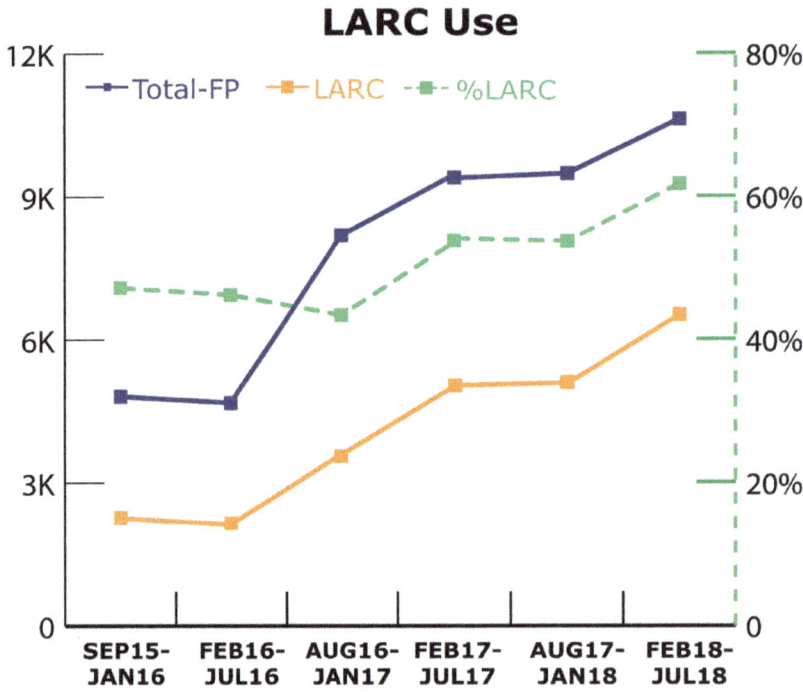

Figure 11. LARC Use by Trimester, September 2015–July 2018

These service data summaries were collated from data collected as part of the routine practice of each of the partnering institutions, with mandates to report to their respective regional health bureaus and/or the FMOH. UM-CIRHT site coordinators and the M&E team played a supportive role, helping identify gaps in collected data and pointing out any obvious errors monthly. This process attempts to rectify any discrepancies in the collected data, but there might still remain systemic, inherent data quality issues at each institution. In a brief audit to check the validity of the raw data from partner sites, some data elements did not reflect expected patterns. The particular concern was the low reported number of clients using short-acting contraceptives. That data may contain a reporting bias for LARC relative to short-acting contraceptive methods, thereby underestimating total FP use.

Most of the sites do not have an electronic database. The paper-based recording and manual reporting methods increase the risk of data-entry errors. This situation is not unique to the partner institutions or Ethiopia but is reflective of systemic infrastructure gaps common to many low-resource settings that go beyond the scope of this program. Over the five-year project, however, the methods for data collection and compilation have improved. The FMOH has data-quality initiatives planned for the coming year that may alleviate this problem in the future.

For all of the FP/CAC services, it is important to note that none of the partner schools had quotas for the uptake of specific services. Success was determined by the access, availability, and range of choices of FP/CAC services for patients.

The design of the Michu clinics as model clinics for FP/CAC service provision provided valuable training experience in bedside care for students and residents. The structure of

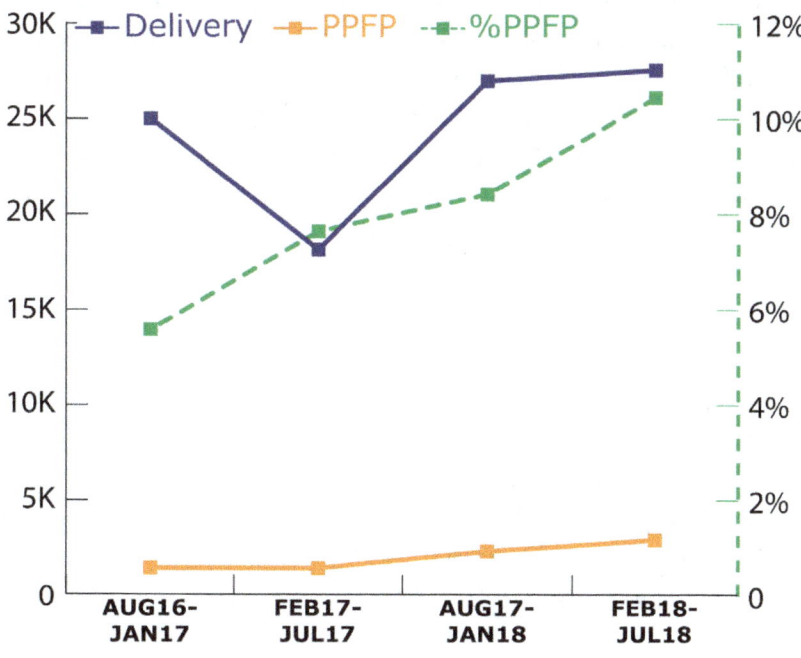

Figure 12. PPFP Services across Partner Schools, August 2016–July 2018

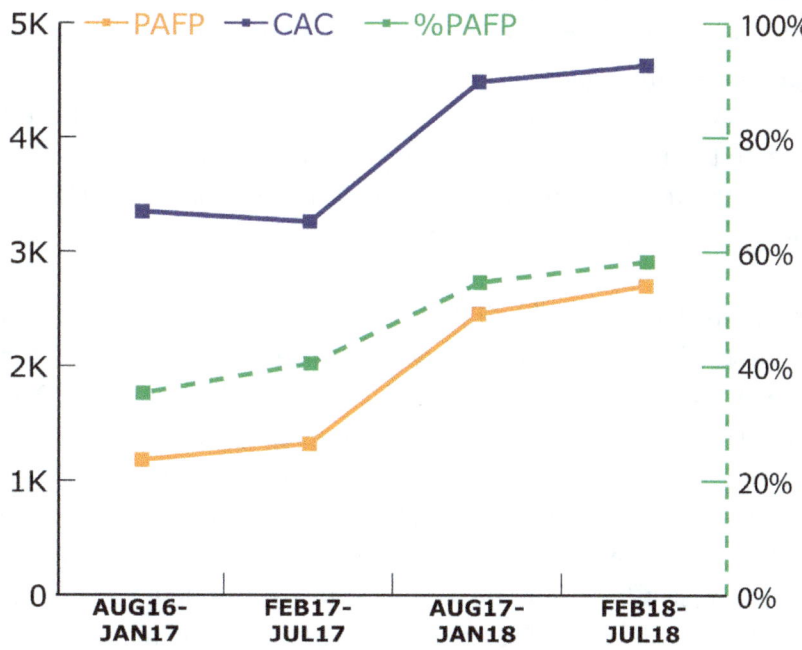

Figure 13. PAFP Services across Partner Schools, August 2016–July 2018

the model clinics challenged the mind-set that FP was only for lower-level providers and provided an alternative model where midwives, nurses, general physicians, and OBGYNs all had a role in FP/CAC counseling and service provision. One interviewee commented on the culture shift in making FP/CAC an interprofessional activity and bringing together *"people who worked next to each other but not with each other."*

The frequency and quality of FP/CAC counseling for patients increased from the initial baseline. Interviewees noted, though, that one side effect of the Michu clinic organizational structure was inconsistency in counseling. The clinics relied heavily on a small core team of providers and the students rotating through them. There was noted variation in the level and quality of services provided, such as how counseling was delivered and who was available to do surgical abortion, particularly in the second trimester.

The clinical service part of the program included training and outreach in professionalism and ethics around service provision for the full range of FP/CAC. It raised awareness of FP beyond providers, including guards and cleaners at hospitals, hosts of radio programs, and policy makers. One UM-CIRHT staff member commented, *"The Michu clinic brought outpatient safe abortion for the first time [to] these teaching hospitals. One of my proudest moments was hearing an OBGYN resident at one of the partner schools speak about CAC to a visiting physician from another country. He spoke about how he changed his perspective toward abortion. He said, 'I now realize, you can have religion and you can do an abortion.'"*

While all partner schools showed an increase in FP/CAC services, the client load at the Michu clinics was still relatively small. As the teaching hospitals associated with the partner schools were all major general or referral hospitals, patients often did not consider them the first option for FP/CAC services. PPFP across the partner schools varied. In phase 3, the FMOH team is planning more PPFP counseling as part of antenatal care.

Through the service program, the partner schools incorporated formal QI methodologies to assess and address gaps in the provision of FP/CAC. This led to improvements in data quality as well as service quality. The QI activities fostered a culture of woman-centered respectful and compassionate care broadly and especially in the sensitive topics of FP/CAC. One interviewee commented, *"There is a lot of learning in Michu clinic, which other countries could also use to adapt to their own model of patient-friendly care for their culture."*

During the transition phase, the FMOH continued training in surgical abortion, QI, counseling, and VCAT. Between August and December 2018, the FMOH team coordinated with UM-CIRHT for on-site training in dilation and evacuation (D&E) surgical abortion at the University of Gondar and Adama Hospital Medical College. They also facilitated an experience-sharing visit where five providers from Gondar visited the St. Paul's Hospital Millennium Medical College Michu clinic to observe D&E cases. During this period, QI committee meetings and projects continued at eight of the nine partner schools. The QI projects included infection prevention training, patient-centered RH service training, basic FP training for newly assigned Michu clinic staff, and RH commodity management training. The QI activities at the ninth partner school are expected to resume in 2019. The FMOH arranged VCAT training for six of the partner schools. Topics addressed included ethics in reproductive health, client-centered contraception, and quality contraception counseling. In 2019, the trained faculty are expected to cascade the information to their respective schools. Additionally, in response to the increased but still relatively small number of clientele at the Michu clinics relative to national FP services, the FMOH plans to increase awareness through PPFP information outreach in antenatal clinics.

### Research

When the research program for OBGYN was launched in June 2015, faculty proposed a total of 185 research topics. These were reviewed by the UM-CIRHT research team for their merit and relevance according to set criteria. Based on this feedback, 39 were turned into full proposals and presented nationally in Addis Ababa to experienced research reviewers from universities and experts from the FMOH. From those 39, 26 were selected for pilot grants and coached through the rest of the research process. Nine of the projects were presented and included as abstracts at international conferences. Twenty-one resulted in manuscripts, of which five are pending journal decisions and another seven published their work in journals.[8, 9, 10, 11, 12, 13, 14] Across all the OBGYN research projects, a total of 247 investigators were involved, including the PIs, coinvestigators, residents, and other research team members. Among the OBGYN projects, there were four multisite research projects led by OBGYN faculty at the partner schools and done in collaboration with the UM-CIRHT research team. By the end of the implementation phase, one was published and the other three were in the data-collection stage.[15]

When the research program for midwifery was launched in February 2017, faculty proposed a total of 374 research topics. These were reviewed by the UM-CIRHT research team for their merit and relevance according to set criteria. Based on this feedback, 42 were turned into full proposals and presented nationally in Addis Ababa to experienced research reviewers from universities and experts from the ministry of health. From those 42, 27 were selected for pilot grants and are being coached through the rest of the research process.

Figure 14 shows the research milestones for both OBGYN and midwifery up through December 2018.

At the start of the transition to the FMOH, the OBGYN research projects were mostly in the manuscript phase, but the midwifery projects were still in the data collection stage, since the midwifery research program started later. Therefore, the FMOH chose to focus its research support on the midwifery projects. The FMOH team did hands-on training through the research advisory council (RAC) in the maternal and child health (MCH) directorate of the FMOH.

The mixture of networking, pilot grants, and training was effective in strengthening the culture of research at the partner schools. Though faculty did not have protected research time, the pilot grants provided an alternate incentive for devoting time to it.

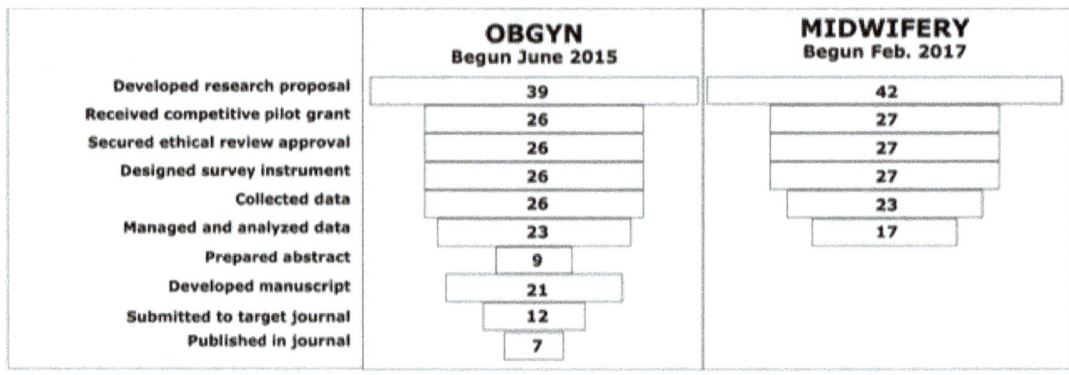

Figure 14. Research Milestones Progress across Partner Schools, June 2015–December 2018

Interviewees noted an invigoration of interest in doing research. Through the project, over 90% of all midwifery faculty across the eight partner schools were involved in one of the research teams. Faculty in both OBGYN and midwifery remarked that they saw an increase in interest in conducting research. They also acknowledged greater awareness and interest among residents in pursuing a career within academic medicine and becoming physician-researchers.

The collaborative approach to research had spillover effects into other departments. The team-science requirement for the pilot grants brought together multiple health sub-specialties and other sciences. The workshops were open to all, not just those with pilot grants. Some PIs who were not selected for pilot grants later joined other teams as coinvestigators. The multisite studies connected people from multiple schools to work together to produce scholarly research at the national scale, formalizing and strengthening existing casual professional relationships.

The alignment of training and implementation with the research life cycle led to a large volume of research projects and resulting manuscripts in a relatively short time span. Interviewees noted that the research writing training addressed a noted skills gap in writing a manuscript with the level of rigor expected by high-impact international journals. This support increased PI confidence in seeking publication opportunities in national and international journals and in sharing this evidence with policy makers.

### Faculty Development

Throughout the initiation and implementation, UM-CIRHT arranged faculty development for education (including leadership), service, and research across all nine partner schools (see figure 15). A total of 174 training sessions were conducted for midwifery and OBGYN: 28 in education, 90 in service, and 56 in research. These training sessions totaled 4,316 contact hours.

Perhaps the most important lesson learned in faculty development was the importance of tailoring the topics to each school and department based on need, availability, and capacity. Through the mix of in-country project staff and advisors across Ethiopia and UM-CIRHT's professional network, the project was able to match experienced instructors with the topics and timing requested by the institutions. Additionally, the inclusion of staff specialists as cofacilitators from the school hosting a particular training demonstrated that the schools had the internal expertise to continue and cascade the training.

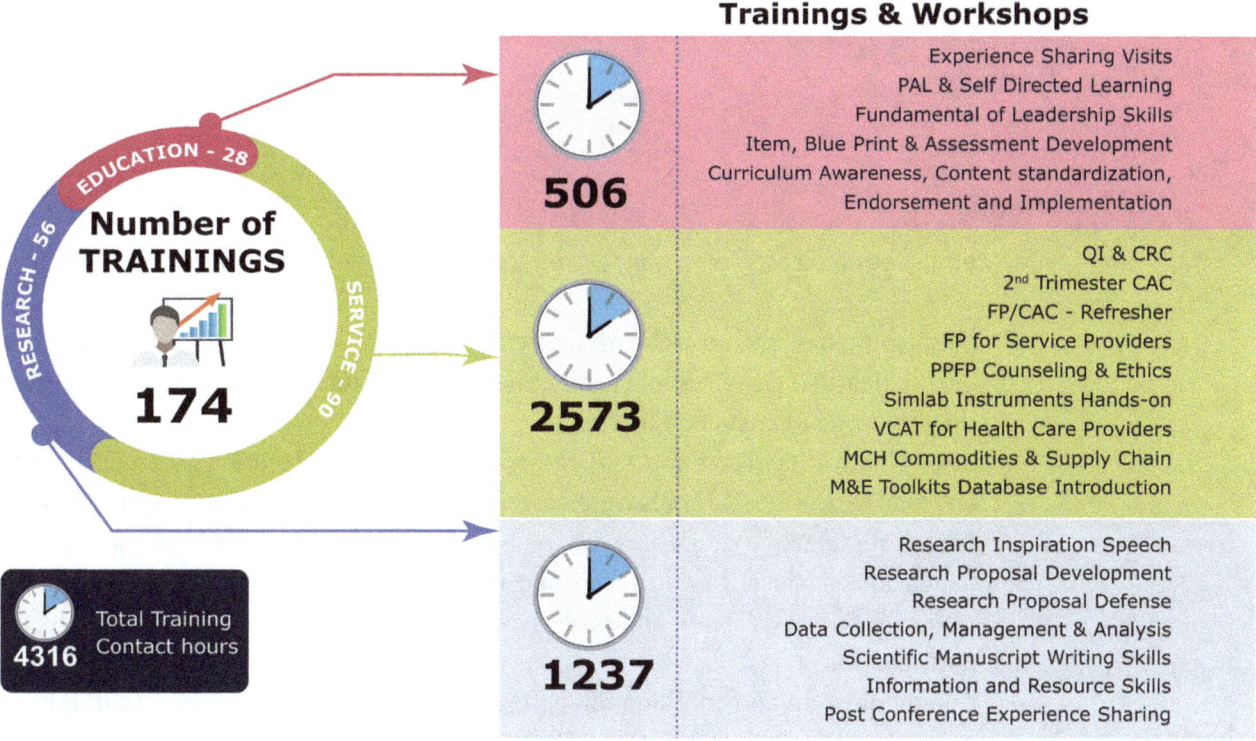

Figure 15. Faculty Development Training across Partner Schools, July 2014–July 2018

## Lessons

### Overall

The interviewees indicated common factors that contributed to the project's success:

- The alignment of the project with the Federal Ministry of Health (FMOH) strategy for overall health outcome improvement helped focus implementation and increased the likelihood of sustainability.
- Strong institutional commitment and ownership of family planning/comprehensive abortion care (FP/CAC) goals were crucial for adherence to educational changes and overall sustainability.
- Landscape analysis of education and clinical infrastructure was helpful; inclusion of business systems and processes landscape analysis is planned for future partnerships.
- Communication and coordination across partner schools were important in planning the curriculum changes.
- Employees worked better as a team when there was clarity of roles and responsibilities.
- Flexibility was key when planning faculty development. Staff worked with faculty to create schedules conducive to other responsibilities, which fostered mutual trust and respect with the partner schools.
- Site coordinators played a crucial role. Employed by Center for International Reproductive Health Training at the University of Michigan (UM-CIRHT) but based at their respective partner schools, they were the nexus between the partner schools and the UM-CIRHT project office in Addis Ababa.
- The preestablished social networks of a large number of stakeholders meant that in many cases, trust and communication were already established.
- Clearly defined shared goals focused work with stakeholders and fostered a sense of energy and enthusiasm within the project.
- The equitable approach to partnering earned UM-CIRHT a generally positive reputation, making new and potential partners eager to join the project.

- Staffing within UM-CIRHT was an important component. Specialized teams and little turnover allowed for consistency in on-the-job mentoring and other forms of technical support.
- The team's response to participant opposition to value clarification and attitude transformation (VCAT) was crucial. They transitioned to an ethical and legal approach, which was received more positively.
- The general approach and attitude of leadership (e.g., provosts, department heads) influenced the attitudes of residents and faculty toward CAC. If school leadership supported FP/CAC, project implementation ran smoothly. If not, providers resisted implementation.
- Monitoring and evaluation (M&E) was an integral part of implementation. Consistent data and data audits over time provided evidence of which interventions were working and why or why not.
- Project management varied with such a large network and scope. The team took a more agile and adaptive approach rather than a tightly controlled, predictive one.

### Education

- Competency-based education (CBE) was an objective way to apply learning goals through simulation and multiple assessment methods.
- Effective coordination with national stakeholders was paramount for achieving a standardized curriculum and core syllabi across all partner schools.
- Curriculum integration required rigorous and consistent follow-up through faculty mentoring and M&E to ensure that the revised curricula and content of faculty development training were translated into practice.
- Faculty and school leadership needed to provide consistent support for the implementation of simulation-based education. This took the form of space, staff, supplies, and so on.

### Clinical Service

- The Michu clinics provided students with model environments in which to experience all levels of provider participation in FP/CAC counseling and services, challenging the idea that FP was only for lower-level providers and showcasing an alternative model.
- The inclusive approach to training and outreach in professionalism and ethics around service provision for FP/CAC raised awareness of FP beyond providers, including among hospital guards and cleaners, policymakers, and so on.
- The incorporation of formal quality improvement (QI) methodologies to assess and address gaps in the provision of FP/CAC led to improvement in data quality as well as in service quality.
- QI activities fostered a culture of women-centered, respectful, and compassionate care, especially in the sensitive topics of FP/CAC.

### Research

- The combination of milestone-based research methodology training, competitive pilot grants, mentoring, and networking was effective in strengthening the culture of research at the partner schools.
- The collaborative team-science approach to research had spillover effects into other departments beyond obstetrics and gynecology (OBGYN) and midwifery.
- The alignment of training and implementation with the research life cycle led to a large volume of research projects, resulting in the development of many manuscripts in a relatively short time span.

### Faculty Development

- To be more effective, faculty development must have focused competencies that focus the training.
- Specification of core competencies for each training topic is helpful for setting trainee expectations and learning objectives.
- The inclusion of faculty or staff from the partner schools as cofacilitators for various trainings increased the likelihood that the schools would have the internal expertise to continue and cascade the training.

## Conclusion

Across the four programs of support, the project significantly benefited the OBGYN and midwifery departments of the partner schools and had a spillover effect on other departments and schools across the universities. This diffusion was visible in research, simulation-based training, and medical education. Through a systematic, phased approach, the project stimulated research interest in relevant RH issues and built the research capacity of Ethiopian faculty while bolstering an authentic partnership between U-M and Ethiopian medical and midwifery schools. One salient feature consistently highlighted by interviewees was UM-CIRHT's unique approach, which has variously been described as nonprescriptive and driven by the needs of partner schools in an authentic partnership model.

The simulation lab renovations and upgrades were highlighted by many interviewees as a significant achievement of the project. While other organizations had done prior work in these spaces, the partner schools credited this project as taking that work to full scale. By designing instruction guides / checklists for students practicing on simulators, the project made it so that students were better able to take advantage of the additional physical resources like high-fidelity simulation equipment. One interviewee commented, *"The simulation equipment is extremely valuable and would have been practically impossible to secure had UM-CIRHT not supported it."* The simulation labs have substantially enhanced the educational programs and are noted as important contributions in teaching the rising number of medical and midwifery students.

One of the goals of this project was to have a national-scale impact on FP/CAC across Ethiopia. The receptiveness of FMOH to lead phase 3 of the project demonstrates the government's strong commitment to continuing and scaling the work initiated during the project. Because of the early involvement of the FMOH in designing some of the programs and the coincidental transition of two former UM-CIRHT employees into FMOH leadership positions, the FMOH is well-informed of the background and poised to continue the work.

One interviewee from the FMOH commented, *"One of the largest successes [of the project] was bringing the FP agenda to preservice. There is a predominant assumption that graduated physicians and midwives are skilled on FP, but they are not. Preservice before had not been able to equip them with sufficient skills. In-service training was necessary to address resulting gaps. UM-CIRHT has changed that cycle."* An interviewee who had served as a faculty champion for one of the partner schools summarized, *"This is a cost-effective method of teaching and learning. I strongly recommend that this approach be scaled up to other medical schools in our country or in other countries."*

## References

1. United Nations. (2015). Sustainable development goals (SDGs). https://sustainabledevelopment.un.org/. Accessed April 30, 2019.
2. Women Deliver. (2019). Meet the demand for contraception and reproductive health. https://womendeliver.org/deliver-for-good/infographics-3/.
3. John Bongaarts and Karen Hardee. (2017). The role of public-sector family planning programs in meeting the demand for contraception in sub-Saharan Africa. *International Perspectives on Sexual and Reproductive Health* 43 (2): 41–50.
4. Lia T. Gebremedhin, Balkachew Nigatu, Delayehu Bekele, Senait Fisseha, and Berhanu G. Gebremeskel. (2016). Integrating family planning into medical education: A case study of St. Paul's Hospital Millennium Medical College (SPHMMC), Addis Ababa. https://quod.lib.umich.edu/c/cirht/mpub9712319. Accessed April 30, 2019.
5. Leontine Alkema, Doris Chou, Daniel Hogan, Sanqian Zhang, Ann-Beth Moller et al. (January 30–February 5, 2016). Global, regional, and national levels and trends in maternal mortality between 1990 and 2015, with scenario-based projections to 2030: A systematic analysis by the UN Maternal Mortality Estimation Inter-agency Group. *Lancet* 387 (10017): 462–74. https://doi.org/10.1016/S0140-6736(15)00838-7.
6. Ethiopia Central Statistical Agency. (2016). Ethiopia—demographic and health survey 2016. http://microdata.worldbank.org/index.php/catalog/2886.
7. Solomon W. Beza, Bekalu M. Chekol, Munir K. Eshetu, Lia T. Gebremedhin, Berhanu G. Gebremeskel et al. (2018). The UM-CIRHT framework for integrating comprehensive contraception and abortion care competencies into health professions education. http://hdl.handle.net/2027/spo.mpub11305653. Accessed April 30, 2019.
8. Million Teshome, Zenebe Wolde, Abel Gedefaw, Mequanent Tariku, and Anteneh Asefa. (2018). Surgical informed consent in obstetric and gynecologic surgeries: Experience from a comprehensive teaching hospital in Southern Ethiopia. *BMC Medical Ethics* 19 (38). https://doi.org/10.1186/s12910-018-0293-2.
9. Fikru Abebe, Ephrem Mannekulih, Abebe Megerso, Abdurahman Idris, and Tsegaye Legese. (2018). Determinants of uterine rupture among cases of Adama city public and

private hospitals, Oromia, Ethiopia: A case control study. *Reproductive Health* 15 (161). https://doi.org/10.1186/s12978-018-0606-4.

10. Yeshiwas Abebaw, Solomon Berhe, Solomon Mekonnen Abebe, Mulat Adefris Woldetsadik, Abebaw Gebeyehu et al. (2019). Providers' knowledge on postpartum intrauterine contraceptive device (PPIUCD) service provision in Amhara region public health facility, Ethiopia. *PLOS ONE* 14 (4). https://journals.plos.org/plosone/article?id=10.1371/journal.pone.0214334.

11. Elfalet Fekadu, Getachew Yigzaw, Kassahun Alemu Gelaye, Tadesse Awoke Ayele, Tameru Minwuye et al. (2018). Prevalence of domestic violence and associated factors among pregnant women attending antenatal care service at University of Gondar Referral Hospital, Northwest Ethiopia. *BMC Womens Health* 18 (1): 138. https://bmcwomenshealth.biomedcentral.com/articles/10.1186/s12905-018-0632-y.

12. Yibiteltah Siraneh and Adhadu Workneh. (2019). Determinants and Outcome of Safe Second Trimester Medical Abortion at Jimma University Medical Center, Southwest Ethiopia. *Journal of Pregnancy.* Vol. 2019, Article ID 4513827. https://doi.org/10.1155/2019/4513827.

13. Sisay Teklu Waji, Amaha Gebremedhin, Dawit Worku, Alula Teklu, Fikru Abebe, Godana Jarso, Kissi Mudie, Tamrat Endale. Risk factors for megaloblastic anemia related hematologic disorder among pregnant mothers attending ANC in eastern Shoa zone and the vicinity. A case control study. *Ethiopian Medical Journal* 57 (2). http://emjema.org/index.php/EMJ/article/view/1130/.

14. Million Teshome, Zenebe Wolde, Abel Gedefaw, Anteneh Asefa. (2019). Improving surgical informed consent in obstetric and gynaecologic surgeries in a teaching hospital in Ethiopia: A before and after study. *BMJ Open*, 9(1). https://doi.org/10.1136/bmjopen-2018-023408.

15. Berhanu G. Gebremeskel, Alula M. Teklu, Lia T. Gebremedhin, Solomon W. Beza, Tegbar Yigzaw et al. (2018). Structured integration of family planning curriculum: Comparative assessment of knowledge and skills among new medical graduates in Ethiopia. *Contraception* 98 (2): 89–94. https://doi.org/10.1016/j.contraception.2018.04.001.

www.ingramcontent.com/pod-product-compliance
Lightning Source LLC
Jackson TN
JSHW052242110426
100741JS00006B/30